Communicating Cancer

Communicating Cancer

Strategies for You, Family, and Friends

Lisa M. Coutu, Ph.D.

Communicating Cancer:
Strategies for You, Family, and Friends

By Lisa M. Coutu, Ph.D.
 Published 2026.

Available via IngramSpark
communicatingcancer.com

ISBN 979-8-9990820-1-5

For Dan, for everything

Lisa M. Coutu holds an M.A. and Ph.D. in the Ethnography of Communication, an area of study where anthropology and linguistics meet. She is a Teaching Professor Emeritus in Communication at the University of Washington in Seattle.

Diagnosed with breast cancer in 2014, at 47 years old, Lisa has been NED (no evidence of disease) since her initial treatment ended. Her natural tendency to look at the world through the lens of communication helped her manage and navigate her experience with breast cancer.

Lisa is doing everything she would've missed if it weren't for her successful breast cancer treatment. She fills her days connecting with family and friends, playing outdoors, being creative, and reveling in her good fortune.

Happily married to Dan Nichol for over 30 years, they live in the state of Washington, where they enjoy their retirement. She knows she is lucky.

Acknowledgements

I am grateful for the community who supported me during both my cancer treatment and the writing of this book. Every person who stepped toward me with love and care during my cancer experience made a difference in my life. Thank you.

Dan Nichol, thank you for being my person, for building me up when I am down, and for rejoicing with me when I am at my best. You encouraged me to write this book, even though the sadness it brings me to revisit my cancer experiences affects you too. Your support buoyed me during my darkest times. I love you, and our life together is my favorite place to be. Your proofreading skills are an unexpected marriage perk—thank you for doing the first close reading of the entire book manuscript.

Thank you Mom (Jane), Dad (Jerry), Jeff, and Darlene Coutu; Catie Coutu Fernandez; and Trish Nichol. You always have my back and celebrate me in ways that make my heart happy. You held me up during my cancer treatment and cheered me on as I wrote this book. I am thankful every day that you are my family.

Thank you Anita Verna Crofts, Dan Crofts, and Jessica Esch for encouraging me to believe in the possibility of publishing this book. Your persuasive nudges brought me back to this manuscript with renewed faith in its potential to help people.

Jessica Esch, I could not have published this book without you. You took my words and magically transformed them into this book. Your keen eye, sharp mind, and well-timed wit helped me bring this book to life. Let's find a lighter topic for the next book, okay?

I appreciate my wide circle of generous friends. Whether you have been with me for decades or for a few short years, my life is richer and more joyful for having you walk alongside me. A special shout-out to Cindy Wright for literally walking beside me for years, listening to me process my cancer experience, this book, and life. I look forward to our next walk.

My "raggedy love army" formed a circle of support and love

around me as I learned to live life with a cancer diagnosis. I still carry you in my heart.

Thank you to the women of Team Survivor Northwest, who helped me find my way back to being healthy and fit.

Thank you to everyone at Swedish Cancer Institute, from medical staff to reception staff, for the care and compassion you have shown me since my diagnosis. I am grateful beyond measure for you.

Thank you to the University of Washington and the Department of Communication for the sabbatical that afforded me the time to write the first draft of this book. And thank you again to Anita Verna Crofts and Trish Nichol for reading and providing helpful comments on the final draft before I submitted this book for publication.

Most of all, thank you all for the love. It's really all that matters to me in the end.

Table of Contents

Prologue

I wrote this book in 2016, shortly after I completed my cancer treatment. At the time, I was a Teaching Professor in Communication at the University of Washington. I sent book proposals to several publishers, but did not ultimately find a place to publish my manuscript. I simply didn't have the capacity to continue pursuing publication while also carrying my responsibilities as a faculty member.

Over the years, the reasons the publishers declined to publish my manuscript continued to bother me. Their bottom line was that there wasn't a market for the book, with one publisher writing:

> *I think a guide to talking with others (including healthcare personnel, etc.) is a great approach to the topic, and incorporating actual communications strategies that are based on academic communications studies is fine. But putting some of the theory and practice into the work makes it less palatable to general readers. They want the strategies, but they may not care about what all the theory behind it is or what all of the research shows—some of the research, yes, but overall the feel here is that the focus is on what the research shows.*

Another publisher suggested that I needed to better target my proposed audience of women with breast cancer:

> *If the primary market is women with breast cancer, you might want to dial back the sections on communication theory, as that audience won't be likely to care as much about that—they will be concerned only with how these theories affect them and their experience.*

As a woman who had breast cancer, I do not want someone to just tell me what to do. I want an expert with credentials and references to give me options. I want someone to tell me where she got her ideas and to be transparent about how I can read the materials that shaped her suggestions. I give us more credit than either of these publishers did.

Since 2016, I have shared drafts of these chapters with others. Recently, I shared the entire manuscript with a friend whose friend was recently diagnosed with breast cancer. He, a well-published nonfiction author, said he thought my book should be published and suggested that it was a book not only for women with breast cancer, but also for the people who care about women with breast cancer. I decided, with the strong encouragement of two dear friends, to self-publish.

As I started to edit my manuscript, my goal was clear—to get this manuscript into your hands, where it may prove to be helpful. In all of my reading of personal breast cancer memoirs and published breast cancer studies, I have not found anything that specifically focuses on how to help women deal with the communication challenges of their breast cancer experience. By communication challenges, I mean not only in healthcare interactions, but also in family, friend, and partner relationships. Our breast cancer is not just about our breasts; it's about our life. And having concrete communication guidance for something most of us never expected to experience can be invaluable.

In the spirit of expediency, I chose not to review the literature that has been published since 2016, except in places where I was concerned that there might be significant changes in our understanding of breast cancer and communication. For instance, I included a recent research article on lesbian couples because most of the research has focused on heterosexual couples. I also checked to make sure that factual information included here is still correct. For instance, I checked to see if the survival rates of African American women with breast cancer were still lower than the survival rates of their White counterparts; unfortunately, that fact remains. I also checked all links to online sources to ensure they still work and that the sites provide relevant information. In general, I kept the format and style the same as it was when I first wrote it, but with editing for readability and usefulness.

So here it is, my book with advice and strategies coupled with research you can judge for yourself. You can dive as deeply as you want into the research by reading some of the materials in the endnotes (many include links to abstracts and/or open source access to articles). Or you can use my strategies as they are, confident that they are grounded in studies of many women like us. Either way, my hope is that my ideas here make your communication with others easier during your breast cancer experience. I offer it to you as the book of advice I wish I had when I was going through the experience myself.

Chapter 1
Introduction to Cancer and Communication

I was on the phone with my mother when the radiologist called me with my biopsy results. I took the radiologist's call, telling my mother I'd call her right back with the results. But how was I going to tell my mother that I had cancer?

Although clearly a physical and medical experience, breast cancer also, very consequentially, involves communication. I have read wonderfully inspiring and honest personal memoirs of women with breast cancer, and many informative academic studies about breast cancer and communication. I haven't found much patient-centered advice grounded in research to help women understand and manage communication during the incredibly distressing experience of breast cancer. Don't get me wrong–there is lots of good advice, but it's mostly based on one woman's experience and what works for her. If you read ten of these memoirs, there will be some overlap, but there is still also much that is idiosyncratic to the individual author's experience. There is also lots of great research on communication and breast cancer, but it's largely written in an academic style that doesn't generally appeal to the general public.

In this book, I tell my story and offer advice, but do so in the context of what communication experts can help us understand about the world we've been thrust into, as well as what we can take from their knowledge to help manage the controllable parts of our new reality. There is so much that is out of our control with breast cancer. One of my mantras during treatment was "control the controllables." Communication, or at least our part in it, is one of those controllables.

I provide research-based strategies for how you can approach your diagnosis, treatment decisions, conversations with care providers, and communication with family and friends, as well as how you can understand the cultural context(s) in which your breast cancer happens. My goal is not to provide one-size-fits-all advice, but rather to provide a range of communication strategies that will empower us to make communication choices in our interactions around our cancer that work best for each of us. I say "us" because I continue to have conversations about and around my cancer, even so many years after my diagnosis. I expect some of these conversations to occur (like the ones with care providers), but others surprise me (like the ones with a new friend who also had breast cancer). I also continue to struggle with my identity and how I convey it to others. In other words, I'm still learning how to do all of this, and writing this book is one way for me to continue to make some sense of and gain control over my world.

Cancer and Communication

You might be wondering what communication has to do with a breast cancer diagnosis and its subsequent treatment. Even as someone who researched and taught communication, it wasn't until a month after my diagnosis, during my first appointment with my medical oncologist, that I realized how much communication was central to my cancer experience. At the end of my appointment, the medical oncology nurse sat down, looked me in the eye, and said, "This is your story. You are the most important person right now. You tell your story your way. If other people start telling you their stories and you do not want to hear them, tell them to stop talking. This is about you. Period." That's when I realized that although "this," the breast cancer, might be about me, "this," the experience of having breast cancer, is about communication.

I admit to a communication bias. It's what I did for a living. I taught and researched communication at the University of Washington for more than 25 years. I mostly focused on how communication shapes, reflects, reinforces, and redefines communities and the individuals who belong to them. Less than a year before my diagnosis, I gave a public lecture at the University of Washington about how my family and personal histories intersected with my academic life. I gave the lecture in the form of a story, noting up front that stories don't just transmit information (although they can do that). They also say something about how the storyteller sees herself, her relationships to others, and the world around her.

So here is my breast cancer story. It says something about how I view myself, my relationships to others, and the world around me.

Like me, you have been told that you have breast cancer. If you're like most of the women I've talked to, there is a clear "before breast cancer" and "after breast cancer" perspective. I'm still the same person, but I'm changed. In retrospect, I managed some of my communication interactions well, and I could have done better in some others.

In 1961, long before the meteoric rise of published breast cancer memoirs, a medical doctor wrote that "the literature on cancer of the breast is too voluminous and too repetitious to review here."[1] More than 60 years later, there's even more to read. There is, in fact, an astounding amount of research on breast cancer and communication alone, much of it produced since the early 1990s.[2] Making research findings accessible and useful to people with cancer is an important part of this work.[3] But there is just so much information that it's mind-boggling. For example, as I began research to write this book, I started by searching my university's library for research articles and books on "breast cancer and communication:" There were nearly 180,000. So, I narrowed my search to "breast cancer narratives," and got 20,938. Then to "breast cancer and couples," and got 42,427. How would I ever get a handle on all of this information to translate it effectively into a helpful form that you and I could use right now? I quickly learned that I wasn't going to get a handle on all of it. I'll draw on relevant articles and books to support my points, but I'm mostly offering you my long-studied understanding of communication coupled with my own experience.

Our communication with other people in our lives changes with a cancer diagnosis. Communication with our healthcare providers is only one (albeit important) part of our communication life around cancer. Cancer can affect us at personal identity, relationship, and community levels. In each of these contexts, communication plays a role. I'll cover these topics in more detail in later chapters, but here are a few examples to illustrate what I mean.

First, when it comes to cancer, and particularly to breast cancer, communication impacts quality of life, quality of care, and quality of health outcomes. The most obvious place this kind of communication occurs is with our healthcare providers. Disparities in treatment and outcomes exist across racial, ethnic, and socio-economic lines. For example, breast cancer incidence in White women is slightly higher than in African American women, but African American women are about 40% more likely to die from it.[4] Many factors may influence the reality of treatment and survival disparities—socio-economic status, tumor biology, stage at diagnosis, poor daily resources, scarce healthcare resources, racism, discrimination, cultural group behaviors and values, individual patient characteristics, and the healthcare system.[5] Communication certainly contributes, as a patient's sense of being able to communicate effectively with physicians has been shown to play a role in whether we follow through with treatment plans.[6]

Physicians are encouraged to consider the cultural and social factors that influence women's treatment decisions and to craft messages in culturally appropriate ways.[7] But physicians and other healthcare providers are only one part of the communication interaction. As women, we can also educate ourselves to optimize communication with our providers so that our treatment is most appropriate and our survival is optimized. Despite the differences in our individual situations, one thing each of us can do is to leverage proven communication strategies to improve our healthcare experiences and outcomes.

People with cancer perceive communication to be connected to their health. In a particularly striking study, every participant "explicitly identified communication as having an impact on their clinical outcome, either positively or negatively,"[8] including their survival. They perceived effective patient-provider communication as beneficial to both their emotional and physical well-being, and ineffective patient-provider communication as detrimental to their emotional and physical well-being.[9] In other words, communication matters in cancer patients' experience of their care.

Second, the communication you have with your primary relational partner can impact both your and your partner's psychological adjustment to your breast cancer, even when you don't spend a lot of time actually talking about your cancer. Specifically, social support, emotional disclosure, and informational cancer conversations have all been linked to either positive health outcomes, increased psychological adjustment, or enhanced relational intimacy.[10] The key point here is that how we talk to each other and what we talk about can contribute to our psychological and physical well-being during cancer treatment.

Third, communication within our families, beyond simply our primary relationship, can also help with adjustment to a cancer diagnosis and subsequent treatment. Women who share their thoughts and feelings about their illness with their family members experience better quality of life and emotional well-being than those who don't.[11] And families who problem-solve in response to a breast cancer diagnosis experience both improved quality of life and improved psychological and physical well-being.[12]

Communication isn't going to cure our cancer, but I propose that empowering women to communicate effectively during our breast cancer experience can increase our quality of life. Why do I say this? Because I believe our communication with each other both reflects and shapes our sense of self, our relationships, and our world. Communication with our loved ones, friends, communities, and doctors, is never neutral. What we say, how we say it, to whom we say it, all matter.

My Story

I am a White, straight, married, child-free woman. I was diagnosed with breast cancer on July 25, 2014, at the age of 47. I can close my eyes and go back to the minute I heard I had cancer. I had a routine screening mammogram, was called back for more images, had a biopsy, and then got the news. I was ultimately diagnosed with Stage 2A invasive ductal carcinoma that had spread to one sentinel node. I had a lumpectomy and sentinel node biopsy, six rounds of Cytoxan and Taxotere, and 35 radiation treatments (including a boost). I took tamoxifen for six years and various aromatase inhibitors for three years. I'll tell my story in more detail throughout the following chapters. For now, though, I want you to know that whether you've just been diagnosed with breast cancer, are in the process of deciding on treatment, are mid-treatment, or post-treatment, I have been somewhere similar. We all experience this disease differently, depending in part on our demographics and our individual cancers, but we also share some commonalities.

When I learned I had breast cancer, it was as though someone flipped a switch and I was a different person. I felt like Alice falling down the rabbit hole, suddenly part of a world I hadn't even realized existed. I used language like this to describe how I felt because I didn't have any other way to talk about it. I reflexively grasped on to what I knew, communication, even though it took me some time to realize I was doing it. What to tell people, when to tell people, how to tell people. What questions to ask. How to filter information. How to respond to people's reactions to my cancer. At times, I felt like I was outside of myself watching myself finding my feet in this new world. I wish I could have coached myself a bit more purposefully. But I did the best I could.

I am not a medico-biological breast cancer expert. If you have breast cancer, you no doubt already have (or soon will have) a team of experts helping you with the medical aspects of your disease. There are also numerous helpful books on the biology of breast cancer and breast cancer treatment. I am also not a breast cancer communication expert, in terms of those who research the myriad ways communication impacts and is impacted by breast cancer in personal, professional, and public contexts. What I am is a communication expert who had breast cancer.

The chapters follow a rough chronology of how I experienced my diagnosis and treatment, but you don't need to read them in order. Each chapter can stand alone, and you should read the one or ones that are most useful to you at the moment. And if you come across a chapter that doesn't resonate with you, skip it. The most important thing to remember is that your cancer experience is about *you*.

Many chapters include communication strategies with a gray background so you can easily find them as well as a few blank, lined pages for you to capture your comments and thoughts as you read.

Chapter Preview

I asked myself a lot of questions during and after my treatment. My questions inspired the chapters that follow.

Chapter 1: Introduction to Cancer and Communication

Chapter 2: Our Cancer Stories

- What's my breast cancer story?
- How do I know what my story is?
- What do I do when my story doesn't mesh with the story people seem to expect me to tell?
- Where do I fit in the world of breast cancer communities?
- What do I do with all of this pink?
- How do I tell people I'm not fighting?

Chapter 3: Our Identity

- How do I wrap my head around having cancer?
- How do I integrate breast cancer into my larger life story?
- How do I integrate breast cancer into my identity?
- How do I manage my identity, verbally and nonverbally?

Chapter 4: Our Communities

- Who do I tell?
- What do I tell them?
- How do I tell them?
- What do I say to them?
- How do I interact with people at work?
- How do I get what I need from my workplace?
- How do I respond to people's reactions?
- What do I do with unhelpful responses?

Chapter 5: Our Healthcare Network

- How do I let my doctors know what I need?
- How do I track everything?
- How do I know if I'm making the right treatment decisions?
- What questions should I ask?
- How do I ask questions?

Chapter 6: Our Relationships

- Why does my primary relationship feel different?
- How do I talk about my physical and emotional changes with my partner?
- How do I talk to my family about my cancer?
- How do I manage the changes in my family relationships since my diagnosis?
- Why do some of my friends step towards me and others step away?
- How do I manage the changes in my friendships?

Chapter 7: When Everyone Else Thinks It's Over

- Why does everyone seem to think I'm done with cancer just because I'm done with initial treatment?
- How do I respond to people telling me that "it's all behind me now?"
- How do I educate the people around me?

Epilogue

Chapter 2:
Our Cancer Stories

I talk a lot in this book about stories and language. Learning about the stories and language around breast cancer helped me understand my reactions to the comments some people made when I told them I had cancer. I felt very uncomfortable when people called me brave or inspirational. I didn't feel brave and I didn't want to be inspirational. I also felt very uncomfortable when people told me that I was strong and that I needed to be positive; again, I didn't feel strong and I didn't always feel particularly positive. Was I going to die because I wasn't brave? Or inspirational? Or strong? Or positive?

Just so we are on the same page, I'm going to provide a short explanation of how I'm using the terms "story" and "narrative." Essentially, a personal story is an individual's account of her own experience. It can be long or short. "I have breast cancer," for example, can be a story on its own. It's a different story than "I'm fighting breast cancer." A personal breast cancer story could also include lots of details about every part of your experience. Larger cultural stories or narratives are socially shared storylines that inform and shape individuals' personal stories.[13] For example, in the United States, a prominent cultural narrative is how, with hard work, anyone can accomplish anything she or he wishes to accomplish. We can hear this cultural narrative in Americans' stories about working hard to achieve their success and assume it applies to everyone. Our personal breast cancer stories are also connected to larger cultural narratives of what it means for a woman to have breast cancer.

When I thought about the language people use to describe breast cancer experiences and how that language connects to larger cultural stories about breast cancer, I began to understand my interactions with people better. I also began to understand that my story about my breast cancer didn't align very well with the larger cultural stories of breast cancer. I knew from my academic studies of culture and communication that cultural stories and language are important because they help us make sense of our world and help us tell our own story. In this chapter, I explain how cultural stories and language can shape, reflect—and sometimes conflict with—personal experiences of breast cancer, and how we can work to take control of our own cancer stories.

Throughout this book, I use relatively neutral words to talk about my own breast cancer. I call it my breast cancer "experience," and I name the medical interventions my "treatment." Some words I don't use are "battle," "struggle," "fight," and "journey." As much as possible, I use literal descriptors like "surgery," "chemotherapy," "radiation," and "process." I do not use imagery-laden terms because they create a persona that I did not embrace during my treatment. I did not see myself battling cancer, fighting to win, or on a journey whose ending I could not predict. My body made cancer; it also had done amazing things for me for nearly 50 years. Although I received a few quizzical looks, I told people I was going to love my body back to health. Because how we talk and what we say matter.

Cultural Narratives of Breast Cancer

The most common cultural narrative about breast cancer goes something like this: We must prevent and, if necessary, fight breast cancer. Early detection is key to beating breast cancer. Women fighting breast cancer are brave, strong, and inspirational. It's important that women keep a positive attitude, maintain their femininity, and don't get beaten down by the battle with cancer. People can support women with breast cancer by buying pink merchandise, wearing pink, and reminding women with cancer how brave they are. In return, the women with cancer should continue the fight and in so doing, will prevail. In the end, breast cancer helps women become better versions of themselves.

This cancer story likely sounds familiar to most people. Maybe even natural. Really, what's the big deal, right? This is just how breast cancer is.

Except, it isn't like this for everyone.

Let me point out some of the ways this story we may perceive as natural is really something we've all created together over time. I'm not looking to replace this narrative with a different one. Rather, I'd like to open up some space for multiple cultural level stories about what it means to be a woman with breast cancer, to make room for people whose perspectives and experiences don't line up with the one prominent narrative currently available as a resource for individual breast cancer stories.

Cultural narratives often include figurative language. Figurative language can be useful because it helps us understand one thing in terms of something we already understand. When it comes to breast cancer, which is an overwhelming and scary thing, using figurative language can help us feel less anxious because the figurative language is familiar language that can help us make sense of the unfamiliar.

A Closer Look at the Cultural Story of Breast Cancer

Here's the story I wrote above again. I highlighted figurative language that provides women with a set of instructions on how to act with breast cancer. In brackets, I included brief comments on what the language means for women with breast cancer.

> We must *prevent* [personal responsibility] and, if necessary, *fight* [battle] breast cancer. *Early detection* [personal responsibility] is key to *beating* [battle] breast cancer. Women *fighting* [battle] breast cancer are *brave, strong,* and *inspirational* [characteristics of women]. It's important that women keep a *positive attitude* [requirements for emotional states], maintain their *femininity* [requirements for physical state] and don't get *beaten down* by the battle with cancer [requirement for emotional state]. People can support women with breast cancer by buying *pink* [feminine] merchandise, wearing *pink* [reinforcing femininity], and reminding women with cancer how *brave* and *inspirational* [social reinforcement of expected characteristics] they are. In return, women with cancer should *continue* [not giving up] the *fight* [battle] and in so doing, will *prevail* [fighting leads to victory]. In the end, *breast cancer helps women* become better versions of themselves [reward for fighting].

Figurative language becomes dangerous when it is dismissed as "just" language. It is not neutral. Rather, figurative language, like the language used to talk about breast cancer, can become so much a part of how we talk about the world, that the connections begin to *seem* natural. What this means for women with breast cancer is that the comparison between breast cancer and war becomes not a way to *understand* breast cancer, but the *reality* of breast cancer. In the following sections, I explore in more detail the dimensions of the cultural narratives around breast cancer.

Personal Responsibility

In breast cancer narratives, we hear images of what it means to be a woman in our culture. Most women I know who have breast cancer have, at some point, blamed themselves for their cancer. What did I do? Did I not eat enough vegetables? Did I not exercise enough? Did I drink too much wine? Should I have not taken birth control pills? Did I give myself cancer? These kinds of questions reflect how our larger society talks about breast cancer. Yes, research shows that good nutrition and exercise can lower the risk for breast cancer, and that hormones in birth control pills may increase the risk of breast cancer. But no one knows for sure why some women get breast cancer and others don't. One thing I've become very clear about: It's not our fault that we got breast cancer.

How many other cancers do you hear people blame themselves for getting? Lung cancer and skin cancer, perhaps, but we don't often hear people blaming themselves for getting colon, testicular, brain, blood, or other cancers. It's bad luck that gives someone cancer and good luck that keeps others from getting it. The self-blame and questioning many of us experience after a breast cancer diagnosis is rooted in larger notions of what it means to be a woman. Specifically, we, as women, are responsible for our lives, and if something bad happens, it's because we did not live up to that responsibility. As if our own questioning isn't enough, other people reinforce our role in getting breast cancer. From the friend who asks, "Didn't you skip your mammogram last year?" to the one who tells you that "Everything happens for a reason," messages subtly blame us for our cancer and not so subtly surround us.

Battle

Much of the language around breast cancer is militaristic. Women fight breast cancer; they win or lose their battle. Cancer is the enemy; we have to use all available weapons to defeat it. Women with breast cancer are brave fighters who courageously stare down their disease. We have to fight breast cancer on all fronts.

This militaristic story line can be traced back to the early 1970s when the U.S. government decided to engage in a coordinated effort to cure cancer, spurred by Richard Nixon's declaration of "war on cancer."[14] Decades later, military language about cancer seems almost natural. There has been enormous progress in treatments for breast and other cancers, but there is still no cure for most cancers. This enemy has proven intractable, even in light of a never-ending supply of troops fighting the disease.

Former President Joe Biden's Cancer Moonshot[15] may shift the way our culture talks about cancer. The idea behind the initiative is similar to the National Cancer Act of 1971[16] in that it promotes better coordination and funding of cancer research at the federal level in an effort to prevent and cure cancers. It remains to be seen if the new language of moon exploration can overtake the very popular imagery of war.

Fate

Another cultural narrative I found among a small subset of my friends was that "everything happens for a reason." A friend said this to me about my breast cancer, and I let it go. The first time. When she said it again, I pushed back. I said that I didn't think that my cancer happened for a reason. She suggested that perhaps God was trying to teach me something and I wasn't listening, so He gave me cancer to get my attention. That I was supposed to learn something through this experience. Or that perhaps because I got breast cancer, someone I know would be motivated to get a mammogram and have her breast cancer diagnosed early, thus avoiding death. I finally said that I understood that she believed that things happened for a reason, but not cancer. The God I know wouldn't give me breast cancer because I wasn't paying attention.

Positivity

There is also a cultural narrative of positivity around cancer generally, and certainly around breast cancer. It goes like this: If you have a positive attitude, you will beat breast cancer. (Notice the military language still present.) This was a particularly hard thing for me to get my head around. To all of the people who hadn't had cancer and told me to "be positive and I'd be ok," I wanted to shout, "How would you feel if someone told you right now that you have cancer?" "Positive" wouldn't likely be the answer. Devastated. Terrified. Panicked. Worried. Angry. Desperate. Those are more likely answers. But it's hard for people to see other people suffering, and so this belief that the sufferers will prevail while smiling through the treatment makes it all easier to manage, at least for the outsiders.

The pressure to be positive exhausted me. I did try to be positive much of the time, mostly for my own sanity, because despair was not a great place for me to hang out. In retrospect, I realized that I limited my contact with people when I wasn't feeling positive. I'm not sure if that's because I wanted people to see me only when I was feeling okay, or if I was daunted by the energy it might take to feign positivity. In any case, it was only later, when people asked me how the last chemotherapy treatments were, that I told people how sick I felt, how much I didn't want to do it, how I preferred to die than face feeling that sick for the rest of my life. Even as I write these things, I feel a sense of guilt, that my words should be more encouraging, more positive. But I think it would have helped me to hear from someone early on that it's okay not to be okay. Having breast cancer is not okay.

Pink

In addition to the words people use to talk about breast cancer, cultural narratives also include visual and action-oriented elements. For example, pink is the color of breast cancer. The color pink paints women as feminine, and its use by marketing and branding campaigns connotes communities rallying against a common disease. Runs, walks, and awareness campaigns show women how to look and feel during and after their breast cancer discovery and treatment.

Many of these campaigns legitimately raise awareness and support for breast cancer research. Others, however, prey on people's desire to support women with breast cancer by encouraging them to buy pink products and services, even though the products or services might very well increase women's risk of breast cancer. It's important for consumers to look critically at the links between the pink products and breast cancer before making purchases that may actually be linked to cancer.[17]

Personally, I did not wear pink at all during my treatment. My bald head, puffy face, and slow gait gave me away as someone with cancer. I didn't want to accentuate those things by adding pink to my look. Others embrace wearing pink, and that's great. You should do whatever feels right to you.

Consequences of Not Adopting the Dominant Narratives

What happens when someone pushes back against the dominant cultural narratives? Communities are invested in the stories they tell about the world, so listeners expect people's personal stories to align with cultural stories. Challenging an important cultural narrative can result in some pushback on the individual doing the challenging. This might come in the form of ostracization, explicit correction, or gentle reminders about what the story is. It can mean that the challenger is characterized as being somehow deficient because of her lack of understanding and acceptance of the dominant stories. Author Barbara Ehrenreich wrote of her attempt to talk about her anger on an online breast cancer forum, only to be met with rebukes for her bad attitude and warnings that she should think positively.[18]

Some people collectively push back against the dominant cultural narratives. Women I met through our shared breast cancer experience wear jewelry and create cross-stitch designs with the words f*** cancer. They give cancer the finger (literally) when one of us dies. They clearly and loudly protest that fighting and having a good attitude don't cure breast cancer, and we have the dead friends to show for it. They also acknowledge and honor that for some of us, the dominant narratives work. It's about doing what works for you, without imposing that on other people.

A set of post-millennial narratives about breast cancer is supplanting somewhat older breast cancer narratives by focusing on the environmental, ethical, and political dimensions of breast cancer causes, diagnoses, and treatments. Although they develop alongside traditional breast cancer narratives, they challenge those narratives by drawing attention to people who die from rather than survive breast cancer, and by engaging "readers and viewers politically, ethically, and aesthetically" through memoirs and photographs.[19]

As much as cultural narratives about breast cancer focus on fighting and winning the battle against cancer with a positive attitude, cancer metaphors cut both ways. In larger discourses about cancer, they are often linked to things that are intractable, hopeless, or invasive. For instance, the Obama administration likened ISIS to cancer, as a disease without a clear cure, but with various treatments that might keep it at bay.[20] Economic systems are likened to cancer, as in "Capitalism is a cancer." If we treat capitalism like we treat cancer, we can suppress it and return the economy to a state of homeostasis.[21] Fear is like a cancer. It spreads everywhere throughout our bodies but can be quelled by courageously recognizing and resisting it.[22]

Dominant narratives pervade our communal conversations about breast cancer. They might resonate with your experience; and they might not. For me they did not. Regardless, it's helpful to be aware of the narratives as you craft your own breast cancer story.

What's Your Story?

Figuring out your story can be hard. My life story didn't include breast cancer and reconfiguring it in a way that made sense to me took a long time. I'm not sure I'm quite there yet. But my story has evolved. The day after I was diagnosed, I sent the following email to a small group of friends and family:

> *I have some difficult news to share. I could really use your support and good vibes. I'd normally talk to each of you, but I just can't do that right now. I'm too emotional, but I'm hoping that if I start the conversation via email, I'll be able to continue it over tea with you :)*
>
> *Yesterday, I was diagnosed with breast cancer. Even writing that sentence seems unreal to me. I don't have a lot of answers to the questions that naturally come with such a statement. All I can tell you is that a radiologist reading my routine mammogram noticed something not quite right and that something ended up being cancer.*
>
> *Love,*
> *Lisa*

I couldn't talk to people for a while. I had no words to describe my experience. Much later, toward the end of my treatment, I wrote the following:

> *I'm keeping my chin up. I've thought a lot about what it means to have a "good attitude" as I've navigated my way through this process. Lots of people have told me I have a good attitude, and that makes me happy—I am trying to stay positive and I hope that it shows.*
>
> *I also wonder sometimes what my options are. If I were reading a book and came across a chapter with my current life situation, I'd probably skip it or, at most, skim it. But I don't really have that option. This particular chapter is in my own life story, so I have to put the book under my arm and keep walking, reading it when I can. I know it will end and I will be on to other chapters soon. But the chapter I'm currently in is part and parcel of everything that came before it and everything that will come after. In the present, it's only one of the story lines of my life; there are others that continue alongside it—my deep love with Dan, my individual and communal connections to family and friends, the value I find in my work, my dreams of learning new things and seeing new places. Cancer is just one small, albeit significant, part of my larger story, and the threads of my experience with it will be*

joined with everything else
that makes me, me.

So, my "good attitude" is
really not so much a good
attitude as it is a
realization, every day,
that this is my life. Good
and bad; easy and hard;
joyful and terrifying.

Love,
Lisa

How I made sense of my cancer developed over time. The language I used to talk about it emerged slowly. I realized early on that a lot of the language other people used didn't really work for me. I didn't feel like I was fighting or that I was brave. I had to find other words that fit better with how I was experiencing my illness. You should adopt the language that feels right for your story. If the words shift through your experience, that's okay too. You get to write and edit your story as you'd like.

As my nurse predicted, people told me their cancer stories when they found out I had cancer. They also told me their friends' cancer stories, their coworkers' cancer stories, their family members' cancer stories. There were so many cancer stories. One person told me that there were two elderly women in his church who had recently had breast cancer, and they were fine, so I'd be fine too. All I needed, according to this man, was a good doctor, a good attitude, and God. He told me this while I was recovering from a lumpectomy and trying to decide which chemo cocktail to have. When I brought up my concerns about chemo side effects, he looked me straight in the eye and said, "You always see the negative in everything." Finally, after he was telling a story about a 40-year-old woman who was dying, I said, "Can you please stop talking about that? I really don't want to hear about women my age dying." He was taken aback, but he stopped talking. I was empowered by my nurse's declaration that I could tell anyone to stop telling their stories. You can too. I only wished I had asked him to stop talking sooner. It was a long night.

Sometimes, other people's stories helped me make sense of my situation. People who were like me in some ways, ways that transcended cancer, usually told these stories. For instance, a walking friend, who became a very close friend since my diagnosis, talked to me about her experience with breast cancer. She told it to help me, to comfort me, to let me know that I was not alone. She did not tell me her story to either minimize or catastrophize my or her breast cancer. She also didn't tell me I had to have a good attitude. I did not have a good attitude when I was diagnosed with cancer, and the pressure to be positive was overwhelming. Was I really going to die if I wasn't upbeat and positive? Seriously? I gathered the people around me who rolled their eyes at the idea that positivity leads to cure, who told stories that buoyed me without being dismissive of my fears, and who had experienced the craziness of a cancer diagnosis.

As you begin to make sense of your own story, a few concrete strategies are included at the end of this chapter to help you get some traction.

Summary

Stories help us make sense of our lives. We tell them everyday in both routine and novel situations. A breast cancer diagnosis, and the story we tell about it, is both personal and communal. Our diagnosis happens to us as individuals, but it is also connected to our society's views of cancer generally and breast cancer specifically. As you weave the reality of your breast cancer into your own life story, you get to decide which parts of the larger cultural narratives work for you and which don't. Remember what my medical oncology nurse said: *This is about you. This is your story.*

Strategies

If a dominant narrative works for you, embrace it!
I mean this from the bottom of my heart. Run with it! Two women I loved died from breast cancer within two years of my diagnosis. One had "be brave" tattooed on her wrist, and her family distributed "be brave" temporary tattoos at her memorial. The other loved pink and wore it with a smile. She was pictured in pink silk boxer shorts, always the fighter, at her memorial. These ways of thinking about cancer helped my friends deal with it. I honored it then, and I honor it now.

Tell your own story.
It's obvious by now that the dominant narratives didn't work for me. If they don't work for you, reject them. Create your own. Find one that does. Change your story whenever you want.

I wrote earlier that I told people I was going to love my body back to health, that it had given me a lot of wonderful years and I needed to help it. I also felt sorry for hurting my body in the way that I did with treatment and I apologized to it repeatedly. This imagined separation between my mental and physical selves allowed me to take care of each in my own way, even though it wasn't the way most people around me talked about cancer.

Think about how you want to respond to people whose comments conflict with the way you want your story to be told.
People called me "brave," "inspirational," and "strong." I rejected these characterizations whenever I had the energy to do so. With a smile on my face, I thanked them for the sentiment, then said: "I am terrified. I am being chased by a herd of wild boars and there is a sheer mountain wall in front of me. I can either do nothing and let the boars overtake me, or I can try to climb the sheer wall. That is not bravery. That is a desire to live."

Take your time.
Remember that this is all about you. You'll find ways of talking about your cancer and telling your story that work for you. In the meantime, be gentle with yourself.

Notes

Notes

Chapter 3: Our Identity

Who Are You Now?

Our identities change along with our stories when we are diagnosed with breast cancer. If you're like me, you struggle with integrating the idea of having breast cancer into a larger story of your life and your sense of self. I asked myself often, "Who am I as a person with breast cancer?" In this chapter, I discuss shifting life stories and shifting senses of self, and how these are shaped by the uncertainty and anxiety that come with a cancer diagnosis. I end with strategies for reducing anxiety and uncertainty, and for managing your identity nonverbally as you interact with other people.

Our life story changes with a breast cancer diagnosis. Not only are we personally transformed, but we must also learn how to tell our story differently, incorporating cancer as a plot line. Sociologist Arthur Frank's work on illness narratives supports this idea that telling stories helps us work out our identities and life story in communication with others.[23] Through reconstructing and telling our stories, we make sense of our experience and our changing sense of self. Communication scholar Shani Orgad's book about women telling their breast cancer stories online reinforces the idea that stories help us make sense of our experiences and identities, and provide a sense of control over our lives during a difficult time.[24]

From the moment someone tells us we have breast cancer, we are living a life interrupted. I searched the phrase "life interrupted" on the internet to see if others had also thought of cancer diagnoses in this way. I discovered a wonderful film called *Life Interrupted* that skillfully captures the stories of 3 women with breast cancer, and in so doing demystifies the breast cancer experience.[25] Listening to their stories helped me think about my own life story and the part that cancer plays in it.

Uncertainty and Anxiety

One of the common themes I've heard and read in women's stories of their breast cancer revolves around uncertainty and anxiety. For many of us, a breast cancer diagnosis arrives with a lifetime of not knowing. Uncertainty and its companion, anxiety, become a new normal part of life. We can manage our uncertainty and anxiety by actively using communication tools, which I'll discuss in this chapter. My uncertainty and anxiety haven't fully gone away, but they ebb and flow over time.

My moments of uncertainty and anxiety have been and continue to be during the periods between specific actions. The time between concrete actions can often be filled with unknowns. For example,

- Between an abnormal mammogram and the follow-up appointment—Why do I need a follow-up?
- Between the biopsy and its results—Do I have cancer?
- Between surgery and the pathology report—How bad is it?
- Between genetic testing and receiving the results—Do I have a genetic predisposition for cancer?
- Between deciding on treatment and starting treatment—What treatment is best?
- Between every scan and getting each result—Is it still there? Has it come back?

Uncertainty and anxiety are not the same things, but they often happen in tandem. For instance, I didn't know what to expect when I was called back for a follow-up appointment after a routine screening mammogram (uncertainty), and I found myself fretting about "what if" I had breast cancer (anxiety). Similarly, I was not sure of my biopsy results until two days after the procedure (uncertainty), and I felt nervous, concerned, and on-edge during that time (anxiety). Breast cancer diagnosis, treatment, and recovery involve moment after moment of uncertainty and anxiety.

I remember, for instance, trying to decide which chemotherapy regimen to follow. I had options, and I had decisions to make. I knew I needed chemotherapy, but there were pros and cons to the various options. During this time, I collected information from a variety of sources, thereby reducing my uncertainty. I read about the drugs being proposed by my medical oncologist; I got a second opinion at another area cancer center; I read some research articles on the drugs' effectiveness; and I learned as much about my tumor profile as I could so that I could give my best guess about how likely it was to return and/or spread. Some of these things that I did to decrease my uncertainty reduced my anxiety; others increased it (for instance, when the second opinion doctors ruled against any chemotherapy at all). When I finally made my decision, my uncertainty was greatly reduced, but my anxiety increased significantly until my first chemotherapy appointment.

Turning Points

One way to get our heads around the impact of a breast cancer diagnosis on our world is to think in terms of turning points. The Oxford English Dictionary defines a turning point as "the critical point or juncture in a process, the course of events, etc., upon which future developments depend; *esp.* a moment at which a decisive change in a situation occurs."[26] Turning points are the life moments when we, our relationships, and/or our view of the world, shift, with a clear *before* and *after* perspective. We experience a variety of turning points in life, many of them directly connected to our communication with other people. With a breast cancer diagnosis, our identity, relationships, and/or view of the world can shift. Understanding turning points and their connection to communication helped me understand my changing sense of self, the world, and my life story post-diagnosis.

I had experienced powerful turning points before in my life, as I am sure you have as well. For instance, at my marriage ceremony, my husband and I were pronounced husband and wife. Before those words were uttered, I was his fiancée, but not his wife. Another example happened when I finished my doctorate. I went into my final oral exam about my dissertation as a student but left a doctor. The shift came when my professor held out his hand to shake mine, saying, "Congratulations, Dr. Coutu." These were happy turning points in my life, moments that called for celebration. I had to adjust my sense of self to being a wife, to being a doctor. In so doing, I also adjusted my life story.

Similarly, I experienced a powerful turning point when I found out I had breast cancer. Even though there was lead up to the moment my life was interrupted, it wasn't until I was diagnosed that I felt my world shift. My breast cancer story starts in June 2014 with a routine mammogram. I left town the day after my screening, only to receive a voicemail from the imaging center asking me to come back for some additional scans. I was out of town for several weeks, so I made an appointment for the follow-up scans for the day after I returned home. The appointment was on July 23, 2014.

My husband planned to accompany me to the appointment, but I told him not to bother. After talking to some girlfriends about their experiences, I was convinced that everyone got called back for additional images so my appointment was no big deal. The mammogram technician did the additional scans and then said that the radiologist wanted to do an ultrasound. I was getting nervous, but I convinced myself that they were just being cautious, and I was grateful for that. After all, there was another woman waiting for follow-up scans with me. This was normal.

After the ultrasound, the radiologist said she wanted to do a biopsy as soon as possible. She had an opening in a few hours. I agreed to wait around, and asked if there was anywhere I could go grab lunch. There wasn't any place nearby, so the radiologist gave me some of her lunch. Uh oh. This didn't seem good to me. Who gives away her lunch?

While I waited, I called my husband to give him an update. I was becoming nervous. When I checked in for the biopsy, the woman I had chatted with in the waiting area was leaving. She was told to come back in 6 months for additional scans, but she didn't have a biopsy. As the ultrasound tech prepped me for the biopsy, I started asking questions. My main question was: What determines whether someone needs a biopsy as soon as possible instead of just follow-up scans in another 6 months? She told me I should ask the doctor.

When the radiologist came in, she said the tech mentioned my question. She described the edges of my tumor as "ratty," and noted that it had its own blood supply. To her, these things were "very concerning." At that moment, I realized that she thought I had cancer. She told me she could call me with the results in two days (on a Friday) or she could forward them to my internist to call me on Monday. I asked her to please call me. I left in a daze, pulled out of the parking lot, and parked on the side of the street. I called my husband. I cried. I told him that they thought I had cancer. On the drive home, I got lost, even though I had lived in the city for over 20 years.

Over the next day, my husband and I decided that he should keep to an already planned trip to another state to celebrate his brother's birthday, even though that meant that he would not be home when I received the biopsy results. We rationalized that I likely didn't have cancer, and even if I did, we wouldn't be able to do anything over the weekend. In retrospect, I have no idea what we were thinking. I asked him later, and he responded that he thought we were both in denial.

The day I was to find out whether I had breast cancer, I hung out with good friends who were visiting from out of town. I remember standing on the sidewalk with them, eating caramels from a gourmet sweets store, as my last moment of joy before my diagnosis. I checked my phone constantly, but there was no call. Finally, at 6pm, sitting on my deck, I called my mom to tell her that I hadn't heard anything and that I'd probably not hear until Monday. The other line chimed in. It was the radiologist. She told me, "I'm calling to tell you what I think you already know. You have cancer."

Looking back at this time, I am struck by how this moment changed my life. It was just a moment. As much as I had sensed that the radiologist thought I had cancer, it wasn't until she called and said, "You have cancer," that my world changed. That moment was the turning point. My sense of myself shifted from healthy to seriously ill; my relationships became more complex (more on this later); and I viewed the world differently, divided into people who had cancer and people who didn't.

Powerful turning points are powerful, in part, because someone's utterance creates an immediate life change. This idea comes from speech act theory, a theory about the way that utterances create, define, and change reality. Language philosophers J.L. Austin and John Searle assert that there are only 5 things we can do with language. Each of the 5 has to do with somehow getting the world and our words to fit, so an utterance either represents the world in some way or shifts the world in some way. In the case of being told we have cancer, the utterance does a bit of both. The words represent a reality, but they also declare a reality. In order for this to work, the words have to be spoken by someone with institutional authority, a healthcare provider. If a coworker told you that you have cancer, you'd probably ignore or reject their statement outright. But when a doctor makes the same statement, we believe that it represents a new reality. Austin and Searle call speech acts like this "declaratives," and use examples like "You are married" or "You're fired" to illustrate how words and the world shift together. For me, "You have cancer" did the same thing. An utterance like this, spoken by a person with the appropriate authority, changes the world of the hearer.[27] "You have cancer" changes us from living in the world of the healthy to living in the world of the sick.

There can also be smaller turning points with a cancer diagnosis.

I remember deciding to get a very short crew cut right after my first chemotherapy infusion, and then to take myself shopping for some fun hats. I've always really liked wearing hats. But every hat I tried on made me look like a chemo patient. And I didn't like that at all. I bought no hats that day. My hair cut was a turning point. Nonverbally, I'd gone from looking like I belonged in the world of the well to looking like I belonged in the world of the unwell. The shift was difficult for me because my identity had not included being unwell until that moment.

Identity

Our identities develop throughout our lives. They are complex and multifaceted. We have a core of who we are, and layers built around that core. Turning points catalyze changes or developments in our identity. While the outermost layers can be relatively easily changed, the core generally remains more stable. Our core identities can include our values (e.g., honesty), cultural characteristics (e.g., religion, nationality), demographics (e.g., race, socioeconomic class), and family background (e.g., interaction patterns, beliefs), all of which are interrelated. Core parts of our identity are difficult to change. Some less core aspects of identity can include beliefs about ourselves (e.g., healthy, strong), our sense of agency (i.e., how much control we have over our lives), and our geographical affiliation. These things can be more easily changed.

Our sense of self can be reinforced and challenged in our interactions with other people. I began to view myself as someone who could and would die. So many people said things like "We're all going to die," or "I could be hit by a truck tomorrow." I found this type of response to my new sense of mortality infuriating. Although it's true that we are all going to die and that anyone could be killed unexpectedly by a truck, these things are true in the abstract. My cancer diagnosis and my awareness of my own mortality were (and remain) concrete.

A more positive instance of a challenge to my sense of self occurred the first time I went to a face-to-face breast cancer support group. We all introduced ourselves, including the stage of our cancer. As part of my self-introduction, I said that I felt bad that I only had stage 2 cancer, while so many other women in the room faced later stages. I didn't feel like I had a legitimate reason to be scared and sad. One of the other women in the group looked at me and said, incredulously, "So, you're apologizing because you don't have cancer bad enough?" My sense of being unworthy of the group's support changed, not only because of what she said, but because she said anything at all.

In addition to the internal, unseen uncertainties of a breast cancer diagnosis, many people also experience physical changes that create uncertainty in their sense of self. There are some physical changes that healthcare providers can predict with amazing accuracy (for example, exactly when my hair was going to start to fall out!). Other physical changes vary by intensity, timing, and whether they occur at all. I experienced hair loss, pallor, weight gain, fingernail and toenail loss, neuropathy, hot flashes, fatigue, sore joints, burned and blistered skin from radiation, loss of sensation in treated areas, mild hearing and vision loss, diminished memory, and loss of muscle mass. Some of these were obvious to everyone; others were/are obvious only to me. The physical side effects of cancer shifted my sense of myself as quite able-bodied to much less so, even though others could not perceive the changes.

Part of our identity involves how we present ourselves to others, the verbal and nonverbal things we do to project a particular sense of self or image. I found it helpful to think about my self-presentation in terms of front and back stage. The terms reflect sociologist Erving Goffman's analogy that life is like theater and we are all actors. We exist both on stage (front stage) and behind the curtain (back stage). We know (whether we know it explicitly or implicitly) that we play different roles on different stages, and that our backstage persona is different than our front stage one(s). I found this to be useful in both thinking about my own self-presentation and understanding how others responded to me on different stages.[28]

These ideas fit into the notion that our identity is complex and multifaceted. "Front stage" is what we show the world—and this might differ depending on who we're interacting with, where we are, what our purposes are, etc. "Front stage" deals specifically with the image we try to project in different social scenes. For instance, I had a front stage persona for interacting with my healthcare providers. I generally tried to be upbeat, matter of fact, and organized when I met with my doctors. I dressed well, arrived with an agenda, and asked questions. I wanted them to see me as competent.

"Back stage" is both the literal and figurative place we can be ourselves, without concern about projecting a particular image. During my chemotherapy treatments, back stage was when I was at home, with just my husband, able to let myself relax and feel however I was feeling. As soon as I left my home or someone visited me in my home, I was on stage, acting as much like my healthy self as possible.

One day, I was out to lunch with a faculty friend on campus. She asked me about my front stage persona rather directly. She remarked that I looked good and asked whether that took work or if I just looked that way. I appreciated her awareness that it might take some work to look okay (because it did). I remember on that day I was wearing an oversized light blue sweater, which I knew went well with my eyes, a coordinating blue hat, my glasses (to mask my lack of eyebrows), and makeup. I was working as hard as I could to not look sick. I realized only much later that my front stage acting had been so good that some people did not know that chemotherapy had been difficult for me.

Managing Uncertainty and Anxiety

I've given you some information about how a cancer diagnosis can impact our identities and increase uncertainty and anxiety around who we are in the world. Engaging in uncertainty and anxiety reduction strategies can help decrease the stress associated with being in the moments of limbo that come with a cancer experience. One of the best ways to reduce uncertainty is to gather information.

We vary in terms of how much information we need in order to feel comfortable. For some of us, more information (and therefore, less uncertainty) may actually increase our anxiety. It's important to think about your own comfort level with uncertainty, and what kinds of things trigger your anxiety. I am an information junkie. I want to know as much as possible. Having information doesn't erase my anxiety, but it doesn't make it worse either. Not having information makes my anxiety level skyrocket. It's important to figure out how much information you want.

One of my relatives who was diagnosed with breast cancer not long after I was diagnosed had a very different information threshold than I have. I met her for dinner after one of her doctor appointments. She was overwhelmed and overloaded by the information the doctor conveyed. My comment to her was, "It seems like you trust your doctor, and you just want him to make the treatment call based on his experience." She said, "Exactly." And that's a totally legitimate approach to managing your care.

There are various sources you can access for a wide range of information about breast cancer. I found different sources of information helpful at different times during my experience. Pick and choose among these sources, bearing in mind your personal information threshold.

Sources of Information

Other Women's Experiences

You may want to learn about other women's experiences with breast cancer. Sources of other women's experience include women's personal accounts of their experience with breast cancer, your family, your friends, and/or your friends of friends. You have a network of people who either have had breast cancer themselves or know other women who have had breast cancer.

The day after my diagnosis, before I was ready to talk to many people, two of my friends' friends called me. They had both had breast cancer, and they understood my situation. They knew how terrifying it was to be immediately post-diagnosis. They offered perspective, guidance, and calm. I also spoke with my cousin, who, just the year before, had breast cancer. She and I mostly laughed, which might seem absurd, but it was immensely helpful. We also cried. A couple of days later, one of my very close friends, with whom I had walked regularly during her breast cancer treatment years earlier, came to see me. We also laughed and cried. Each of these women offered me their experiences in ways that were helpful and supportive to me. I have found women who have had breast cancer to be amazingly generous in talking with newly diagnosed women (and newly post-treatment, and so on!).

You can also find information about other women's experiences on the internet. I am ambivalent about this source of information. On the one hand, interacting with women online—or just reading about their experiences—can be enormously helpful. You have a wider range of people than are in your own network, and you can access them from anywhere at any time. Thanks to a friend, I connected with a private Facebook group of young breast cancer survivors. These women, who I did not meet in person for many months, provided a place for me to ask questions. When I finished treatment and found myself sad and anxious, this group of women validated my feelings and helped me find resources to understand my feelings post-treatment as normal and common. On the other hand, because breast cancer is such a widely variable disease, women have widely variable experiences. The internet can be rife with anxiety-inducing stories from women whose lives and disease may be vastly different than yours.

You can also learn about other women's experiences by joining online or face-to-face support groups. You can find online community information at The American Cancer Society (cancer.org/treatment/support-programs-and-services/online-communities.html), as well as at your treatment facility. Face-to-face support groups may or may not be for you, and they may be for you at some times and not others. These groups can be professionally led or survivor led, can be open (you can come and go) or closed (you join for a particular program), and they can be specific to particular concerns or general. You can find face-to-face support information at the American Cancer Society (cancer.org/treatment/support-programs-and-services/resource-search.html) and Living Beyond Breast Cancer (lbbc.org/get-support).

The Internet

The internet teems with medical information about breast cancer. My internist told me specifically to avoid it, that if something needed to be researched, it was my husband's job to do that. I wish, in retrospect, that I had followed her advice. The information hound in me constantly looked for information, especially when I was anxious, in the middle of the night, thinking about my mortality. Bad idea. Because there is just too much information. And only a small fraction of it applies to each individual one of us with breast cancer.

For instance, I was devastated to learn immediately after surgery that I had stage 2A cancer, instead of stage 1. I dove into the internet, searching specifically for survival rates because, after all, that was my main concern: Would I live? My internist had told me that my initial diagnosis was treatable and beatable. But was this still true? When I brought the survival statistics I found online to my surgeon, she asked me a series of questions about the women in the stage 2A group statistics I was citing: How old were they? How healthy were they generally? What other information did I have about their tumor profiles? I had no answers and she made the point that survival statistics can be misleading because the people they represent have such diverse lives and diseases.

Looking at the internet for information is the one information-seeking behavior I did that increased my anxiety significantly. I have mostly stopped doing it, but I still sometimes search for specific information. I advise you to figure out whether searching the internet increases or decreases your anxiety and then make your decision about this as an information source accordingly. If you do decide to rely on the internet for information, below is a list of some reputable sites to search. Also ask your healthcare providers about reputable sites, as these will shift over time after this book is published.

Reputable breast cancer sites:

- Breastcancer.org is a non-profit organization that provides information with the goal of helping women make informed care decisions. breastcancer.org
- American Cancer Society (ACS) provides information about all aspects and phases of breast cancer diagnosis and treatment. cancer.org/cancer/breast-cancer.html
- National Cancer Institute (NCI) is the U.S. federal government's center for cancer research. They provide information for both patients and healthcare providers. You can contact them to ask questions about anything related to your cancer. cancer.gov/contact and cancer.gov/types/breast
- Susan G. Komen is one of the most recognizable organizations focused on breast cancer. They provide information and financial assistance to women and fund research. komen.org/breast-cancer
- Breast Cancer Action is a grassroots, national, activist organization that challenges the focus of many mainstream breast cancer organizations; advocates for health justice for all women facing breast cancer; and provides information and personal guidance to women making decisions about breast cancer screening, prevention, and treatment. bcaction.org
- Young Survivors Coalition (YSC) focuses on the unique concerns of young women diagnosed with breast cancer. YSC provides information and support (both online and face-to-face). youngsurvival.org/who-we-are
- Living Beyond Breast Cancer (LLBC) provides information and support for women at all points of their breast cancer experience. lbbc.org

There are many other sites devoted to breast cancer, but the ones I've included here focus on providing women with the tools and information we need to deal with our breast cancer. My list is not exhaustive but rather points you to information-rich sites that can help you get your head around your cancer. My hope is that by doing some of the legwork for you, I can help you avoid getting sucked into websites that might be unhelpful or unnecessarily anxiety-producing.

Books

You can also find lots of breast cancer information in books. There are tons of books on breast cancer, some focusing on individual women's experiences, and some focusing on breast cancer from a clinical perspective. Here are some of my favorite books in each category:

- Braddock, S., Kercher, J., Edney, J., Block, M, & Clark, M.M. (2015). *Straight talk about breast cancer: From diagnosis to recovery*. Addicus Books. This book is *about* breast cancer, *for* breast cancer patients.
- Leifer, J. with Leifer, L.L. (2015). *After you hear it's cancer: A guide to navigating the difficult journey ahead.* Rowman & Littlefield. John Leifer is a healthcare consultant. After his wife, a radiation oncologist, became a breast cancer patient, they teamed up to write a compelling and comprehensive patient-centered guide to dealing with every aspect of cancer diagnosis, prognosis, and treatment.
- Lucas, G. (2004). *Why I wore lipstick to my mastectomy.* St. Martin's Press. This compelling, poignant, sometimes funny memoir by a young woman with breast cancer highlights moments ranging from finding a lump, to mastectomy, to chemotherapy, to reconstruction, to posing for *Self* magazine. The best breast cancer memoir I have read.
- Peltason, R. (2008). *I am not my breast cancer.* Harper. Peltason draws on excerpts from a blog she co-created with Marc N. Weiss for women with breast cancer. She includes more than 800 women's voices in the book. The scope of this project is amazing and her highlighting of women's voices is wonderful.
- Port, E. (2015). T*he new generation breast cancer book: How to navigate your diagnosis and treatment—and remain optimistic—in an age of information overload.* Ballantine Books. Port is chief of Breast Cancer Surgery at The Mount Sinai Hospital and co-director of the Dubin Breast Center. She filters the overwhelming amount of

readily available medical information and provides fabulous resources (i.e., facts, strategies, myths, glossary) for women with breast cancer.

- Prijatel, P. (2013). *Surviving triple-negative breast cancer: Hope, treatment, and recovery*. Oxford University Press. Prijatel focuses primarily on triple-negative breast cancer (TNBC) but explains the biology and treatment options for all variations of breast cancer. As a woman with triple-negative breast cancer herself, Prijatel draws on her journalism skills to synthesize the research on breast cancer into a well-written, informative, and accessible book.

Healthcare Professionals

You will no doubt seek medical information. You can get some of this information from the internet and other women with breast cancer, and you may find that helpful. But your breast cancer is unique to you, so medical information from the internet and other women with breast cancer can be tricky. The medical information I found most helpful from other women was about how to deal with side effects of treatment, and what to expect before, during, and after treatment.

The most obvious source of medical information is your healthcare providers. This includes both the healthcare providers you have normally seen and the new ones you meet as you begin and then move through treatment. Within a week of my diagnosis, I had spoken to or met with my internist, my naturopath, and my acupuncturist. My internist, for whom I was a very new patient, gave me clear information about my initial diagnosis. She characterized my cancer as "treatable and beatable." My naturopath, who I had seen for 20 years, helped me understand my options for maintaining my health during treatment, and referred me to a naturopath who specialized in cancer treatment. My acupuncturist (in addition to providing wonderful emotional support) informed me of the role of acupuncture in managing treatment side effects.

You will meet a lot of new healthcare providers. In addition to my internist, naturopath, and acupuncturist, I eventually had a breast surgeon, medical oncologist, radiation oncologist, radiation technologists, physical therapist, cancer psychiatrist, onco-physiatrist (a cancer rehabilitation specialist), and many nurses. Each of these people can be a source of information for you. It may feel overwhelming to think about what questions to ask to whom.

And then it may feel overwhelming to think about processing all of the information you gather. I'm including here a list of all of the questions I asked my healthcare providers during my treatment, including what I asked, whom I asked, and when I asked the questions. I kept a notebook that I carried from appointment to appointment. I wrote down questions and concerns before each appointment, and I wrote down questions and concerns after each appointment to ask the next time. At my major appointments that involved gathering information to help with treatment decision-making, I always had my husband accompany me to take notes and to make sure that I had all of my issues addressed.

I'll have more to say about communicating with healthcare providers in chapter 5, but for now, here are the questions and concerns from my notebook. These questions and concerns are all about gathering information to help you reduce uncertainty about your care and condition. If you are someone who does not need or want more information, skip this section. Reading my list may give you more information than you want, as my questions and comments are unedited and include specific aspects of my treatment experience.

On reflection, my questions and concerns are a lot, but they did ensure that I received the information I needed. I'm sharing them with you so you have a place to start.

My Notebook: Questions & Concerns

Internist (pre-oncology appointments)
- Am I going to die?
- What's the treatment timeline?
- Did I give myself breast cancer drinking wine?

Surgeon (pre-surgery)
- My cancer is in my left breast, but I have a pulling sensation in my right breast. What is that?
- What does the MRI show?
- Taking everything together, what are my surgery options? What are the risks associated with waiting for the genetics results?
- What are the survival, local recurrence, and other recurrence rates for lumpectomy + radiation vs. single mastectomy vs. double mastectomy?
- What are the long-term risks of radiation?
- Can I continue to take calcium? Vitamin D? Iron? Adrenal support?
- What are the recurrence rates with each treatment option?
- How does each treatment affect the 5-year survival rate?

Surgeon (post-surgery)
- What does the pathology report "mean"?
- Looks like the grade is different than the grade from the clinical pathology report…
- Cancer in one sentinel node—what does "focal" mean?
- What about the area in MRI, near the biopsy?
- How does cancer in the sentinel node affect treatment?
- I have some numbness. Will it go away?
- What do you think about diet's influence on breast cancer?
- Can I start yoga next week?
- What are the next steps?
- What about cosmetics ingredients' influence on breast cancer?
- What about regular life—dentist, dermatologist, waxing?
- What about this puffiness I have under my arm?
- What are the recurrence rates with each treatment option?
- How does each treatment affect the 5-year survival rate?

Questions and concerns from my notebook

Medical oncologist (post-surgery)

- How many sentinel nodes do I have?
- Could this cancer be other places, too?
- Should I have any other scans?
- How does cancer in the sentinel node change the chemotherapy approach?
- How does the Z0011 trial change chemotherapy approach, given no axilla dissection?
- What should I expect for my work schedule?
- What is the timing for chemotherapy?
- What's my prognosis?
- Can I get a flu shot?
- Can I take adrenal support?
- What about radiation? Risk to my heart?
- Is there a substitute for Adriamycin that doesn't have possible heart damage risk?
- Is there a medication that can mitigate Adriamycin's potential to do heart damage?
- Do I need to be concerned about my mitral valve prolapse increasing the chance of heart damage? What about my family history of heart attacks?
- Will there be tests on my heart prior to treatment?
- What are the cognitive side effects of chemotherapy?
- Is there a naturopath you'd recommend?
- What do you think about acupuncture?
- What are the recurrence rates with each treatment option?
- How does each treatment affect the 5-year survival rate?
- What diet do you recommend?

Second-opinion oncology team (post-surgery)

- Is any additional surgery necessary?
- What constitutes a negative margin?
- Question about Oncotype DX: The Oncotype DX test is designed for women with lymph node negative results, and for post-menopausal women. So, what does that mean in my case (i.e., one positive node and premenopausal)?

Medical oncologist (after second opinion)

- Do you recommend chemotherapy or no chemotherapy?

My Notebook: Questions & Concerns

Research nurse and medical oncologist (after first chemotherapy infusion)

- I didn't seem to have steroid energy.
- How concerned should I be about the growth in my uterus?
- I got a headache during the Cytoxan (during first treatment).
- Do chemotherapy side effects intensify?
- Can you complete my Family Medical Leave Act (FMLA) paperwork?
- What are your thoughts about a post-radiation beach vacation?
- What about these sensations—are they side effects? Tongue feels funny; hands are itchy; nausea?
- Is it ok to take 14-day Prevacid every day?

For research nurse (after second chemotherapy infusion)

- What caused the bruise on my port?
- I am having a Neulasta site reaction.
- What should I do about the Cytoxan headache?
- I was dizzy.
- I had nausea.
- I had diarrhea. My stomach was bad all week. What can I do?
- I was fatigued until day 9. Is that normal?
- What can I put on my head rash?
- What are the names of the people at the front desk?
- I have vaginal burning. What's causing that?
- Should I stop taking iron?

Research nurse (after third chemotherapy infusion)

- Why do my eyes keep watering? Is there something I can do about it?
- Is it ok to have a Christmas tree?
- Should we move the follow-up blood work?
- Am I taking the dexamethasone correctly?
- What does the doctor think about hysteroscopic surgery timing?
- Why is sex painful?
- I have a stitch poking out of my port incision. Should I do anything about it?
- Can I hang out in a hot tub?

My Notebook: Questions & Concerns

Research nurse(after fourth chemotherapy infusion)

- What can I do about hot flashes?
- I have bad indigestion and heartburn, even taking Prilosec once each day.
- I have back and chest pain after chemotherapy.
- I seem to be waking up gasping, having trouble getting a full breath.
- My port seems irritated.

Research nurse (before fifth chemotherapy infusion)

- My port still seems irritated.
- My fingernails and toenails are lifting off.
- I saw people on Thursday who came down with the flu on Sunday. Should I be concerned?
- What tea do you recommend for hot flashes?

Research nurse (after fifth chemotherapy infusion)

- I continue to be concerned that I didn't have more lymph nodes removed. How confident are you in the Z0011 trial?
- Is there any reason to have my ovary and uterus just removed? Am I at an increased chance of uterine or ovarian cancer?
- Can I have radiation and hysteroscopy on the same day?
- How long after chemotherapy does radiation usually start?
- I really feel like I have to concentrate on breathing the first few days after chemotherapy, especially when I'm trying to fall asleep.
- I continue to have hot flashes, nausea, and exhaustion.
- My nails are getting worse.
- Does my port look ok?

Radiation oncologist (pre-radiation)

- What should the timing of radiation with my hysteroscopy be?
- Is it ok to take multivitamins still?
- What lotions do you recommend?
- What is the range of field to be radiated? Including sentinel nodes and neck? Including booster to tumor area?
- I need to file for more FMLA leave from work, now that I'm having new treatment. Is it reasonable for me to ask for 2 days off per week?

My Notebook: Questions & Concerns

Medical oncologist (before sixth chemotherapy infusion)

- My hysteroscopy is set for XX. Is that ok?
- When do I start Tamoxifen?
- When will my port be taken out?
- How long does it take for my body to get back to normal? Eating? Exercising?
- Will follow-up continue to be blood work? Will there be any scans?
- Why is my pinkie finger swollen?
- I have weird sensations at my fingertips.
- Do you think my port looks ok?

Ob/gyn (before surgery to rule out endometrial cancer)

- Should I use pre-surgical soap everywhere?
- Why kind of anesthesia will you use?
- Why are we doing this? If to confirm that the growth is benign, great; if for bleeding . . . I'm not bleeding anymore. Is that normal?
- What kind of downtime should I expect after the procedure?

Medical oncologist (after sixth chemotherapy infusion)

- Can I consume soy?
- Are there other eating or drinking issues on Tamoxifen?
- Is it ok to travel right after radiation?
- How frequently will I be checked after treatment?
- Can we talk about options to deal with painful sex?
- What is the percentage change of systemic recurrence post radiation?
- Is it ok to have hysteroscopy on Wednesday?

Radiation oncologist (during first week of radiation)

- What is the field of radiation?
- Is it ok to travel right after radiation ends?
- Are you ok that I included the week before radiation started on my FMLA, through the end of April?
- Is it ok to take multivitamins?
- What is the value of B6 and glutamine?
- Why are my fingers swollen?

Questions and concerns from my notebook

Medical oncologist (after end of chemotherapy)
- Are B6 and glutamine curative?
- Can I go to the dentist?
- My hands and feet are itchy. Why?

Medical oncologist (before starting Tamoxifen)
- I had low iron stores going into this. Can we check that so that I know whether that's a part of my fatigue?
- I'd like a copy of my treatment plan/summary.
- What language do I use now—"cured" "in remission"?
- What kind of follow-up will I have? Scans? Blood work? Timing?
- Will my period come back?

Radiation oncologist (after end of radiation treatment)
- My chest tissue hurts.
- I have joint pain.
- My mouth is dry.
- Is there anything I should be concerned with moving forward?

Medical oncologist (at three-month follow-up after end of chemotherapy)
- I have some side effects (dry mouth, aching bones, hot flashes)—are those from Tamoxifen?
- My vision seems to have gotten worse.
- I'm still experiencing peripheral neuropathy.
- I'm not due to have a pap smear until 2019; would you recommend yearly?

Medical oncologist (at six-month follow-up after end of chemotherapy)
- Side effects: dry mouth, burning skin (with sweating), hot flashes, fingernails lifting, fatigue, aching feet, hearing loss, vision loss, shoulder pain, memory issues, depression, sleep problems
- Can I take Claritin D and use Flonase or Nasacort?
- What should I be alarmed or concerned about moving forward?
- Is my port scar healing properly?
- Is it ok to take baby aspirin when I fly or am in remote places (for blood clot risk)?

My Notebook: Questions & Concerns

My Notebook: Questions & Concerns

Medical oncologist (at one-year follow-up after end of active treatment)

- I'm going to Belize and will not be close to a hospital. What should I do about the Tamoxifen?
- I'm having pain on my left side and shoulder.
- I'm constipated.
- I'm still having hot flashes.

How to Manage Your Front-Stage Personae

As your uncertainty and anxiety decrease (and they likely will over time), you will begin to integrate the reality of breast cancer into your life story and identity. As you do this, you can also think about how you want to present yourself to the world when you are "front stage."

Everyone has multiple front-stage personae and it takes energy to manage them. (It also takes energy to deal with people's reactions.) Whether and how you manage your self-presentation is always up to you. You get to decide where you expend your energy. The following strategies can help you actively manage your front-stage personae during your breast cancer experience.

I'll focus on nonverbal strategies here because I cover verbal strategies extensively in chapters 4 and 5 when I discuss how to talk with family, friends, colleagues, and healthcare providers. The visible, physical effects of breast cancer treatment can be striking and can profoundly impact our sense of self.

Some of our nonverbal communication cues are more easily controlled than others. For instance, clothing, make-up, and headwear are all controllable, whereas complexion, hair loss, and weight are harder to control. Every breast cancer treatment has physical side effects. Think about how you want people in the different contexts of your life to see you. Once you have those pictures in your mind, you can make some choices about managing your appearance in a way that works for you.

For example, at work, I wanted people to see me as competent and engaged. Most of my coworkers knew about my breast cancer, but when I was at work, I didn't want that to be the first thing they noticed. When I was out shopping, however, around people I didn't know, I didn't really care what they thought of me so I did whatever felt most comfortable at the time. And, as a final example, when I was out for dinner with friends, I wanted them to see me as the person I'd always been so I tried to look as much like my healthy self as possible. Each of these personas called for different kinds and amounts of attention to my appearance. Below, I offer some suggestions for things you might do to project various identities.

Mastectomy

I have not faced the decisions that you will face if you have a mastectomy. The loss of one or both breasts comes with lots of decisions about self-presentation. Breasts are intimately tied to femininity and sexuality in our culture and similarly can be tied to our individual sense of femininity and sexuality. If you have a single or double mastectomy, it is up to you whether you want to have reconstruction, wear prostheses, have male contouring, get tattoos, or do nothing. If you decide to wear prostheses, you can also choose whether or not to wear them in every setting. One of my friends, for instance, wears her prosthesis when dressed up or at work (so her clothes fit the way she likes), but not when she works out or is hanging out with friends. Some of the book and online resources I mentioned earlier in this chapter would be useful places to learn more about your options post-mastectomy.

Lumpectomy

There are not many outwardly visible signs of a lumpectomy. You will have a scar, but its location, size, and appearance will depend on your cancer and your surgeon. My lumpectomy scar is barely noticeable to me on a day-to-day basis. The thing that surprised me, though, was the scar from the sentinel node biopsy. It is under my arm and it looks like a fat fold. I remember complimenting my surgeon on my lumpectomy, but saying that it felt like she really dug around in my armpit. The scar shows when I wear sleeveless shirts. I opt to think of it as just another fat fold, but could cover it easily by wearing shirts with sleeves.

Chemotherapy

Chemotherapy can result in a lot of physical changes, depending on your treatment. I had experience with a wide range of physical effects and will comment on the common visible ones here.

Central Line

You may have a central line or port through which your chemotherapy is administered. I had not thought of this before my treatment, so was surprised that it had as much of an impact on me as it did. My port was above my right breast and was visible if I wore v-neck shirts or anything snug (which became almost everything as my treatment progressed). I chose to wear crew neck or turtleneck tops to cover the port site. I also often wore loose fitting sweaters or jackets.

Some people choose not to have their ports removed. You and

your medical team decide this together. Whether you choose to remove it or retain it, you can make some decisions about whether your port site is visible to other people. My port site was often irritated, and because of concern with infection, my oncologist ordered it removed two days after my final chemotherapy. I was left with a wide, raised, pink scar that I was very self-conscious about. A year after my port was removed, a plastic surgeon used steroid injections to flatten the scar. The scar faded over time and is now barely visible.

Hair Loss

You may lose your hair. I did. The thing that surprised me is that I lost my hair everywhere and it didn't start with my head! The only really visible hair loss you'll experience is on your head and face. I eventually lost all of my hair on my head and face, including my eyebrows and eyelashes.

You have choices about how to present yourself to the world. I chose to embrace being bald, mostly because I didn't want to hassle with a wig. I wore pretty hats or just went bare headed. I have friends who have worn wigs in some settings, but not others. And I have friends who have used being bald as an opportunity to play around with lots of different wigs. The biggest issue with being bald is that it's obvious to everyone you interact with, so they likely know that you are going through cancer treatment. I was okay with that. It may have made some people uncomfortable, but I was pretty uncomfortable myself.

If you lose your eyebrows and eyelashes, you also have some choices about how to present yourself. I wear glasses, so I often didn't bother doing anything with my eyelashes and eyebrows. But, if I was going to work or out on a date with my husband, I drew on eyebrows. I also tried false eyelashes. You can find false eyebrows and eyelashes on the internet (yes, eyebrows too!). Whatever you choose to do, it's about what makes you feel good about your self-presentation.

Weight Gain

You may gain weight during treatment. I did. I also had a puffy face caused by steroids. Most of my clothes didn't fit the way they once did. I bought a few things that were comfortable so that I could wear clothes that fit my current body. This helped me feel confident and comfortable when I was around people. Shopping for clothes during this time was sometimes traumatic for me because nothing fit the way I was used to, but my goal was to look as put together as possible and to feel as comfortable as possible.

Fingernail Changes

I had some fingernail and toenail changes that surprised me. I ended up with white lines across each of my nails, one line for each chemotherapy infusion. All of my nails eventually lifted off the nail beds so that I ended up with nails covering only about one-third of each bed. I wore fun colored nail polish at all times. Even though professional manicures can spread bacteria, I gave myself home manicures throughout my treatment. Regardless of the front stage context I was in, I wanted my hands to look good. The missing fingernails were not as obvious when I painted the remaining parts.

Complexion

During treatment, I was either very pink from taking steroids or very pale from other medications. I tended to wear makeup when I was at work or out for fun, as I wanted to look as normal as possible. I skipped makeup when I was just out and about. You should make the decision that helps you project the image you want to project. If it's important for you to look as healthy as possible at all times, then you might want to consider wearing makeup.

Other Side Effects

You will likely have other side effects from chemotherapy. However, most of them will not be visible and so aren't really a part of your choices about how to present yourself in front stage contexts. This doesn't mean they are unimportant, just that they are hidden aspects of your treatment. I used to say that hair loss was the easiest side effect to endure because some of the others, though invisible to other people, were much more consequential for my daily life.

Radiation

After chemo, radiation initially seemed easy. It wasn't. I had 28 full breast radiation treatments, and then a 7-day boost to my lumpectomy area. Because my cancer was in my left breast, I had to use The Active Breathing Coordinator™, a device that helps reduce the risk of damage to the heart by using a patient's breath to move the heart away from the radiation beam. After a few weeks of treatment, I was tired and burned. Eventually, I had blisters along my left collarbone. Most of my burns were not visible to anyone, but I had to dress strategically to hide both the collarbone burns and the fact that I could not wear a bra because of the burns. Loose clothing that covered most of my chest area allowed me to function without most people seeing my burns.

Bottom Line

You have options. You get to decide how you present yourself to the world during treatment. There is no right answer. It's also important to remember that even with your best efforts, you may not project the image you hope to project. I was devastated one day when a work acquaintance and I were talking after a meeting, and she kept referring to "Lisa." She didn't recognize me! And I thought I looked pretty good. When I finally said, "Mary, it's me. I'm Lisa," she asked, "Oh, I didn't recognize you. Have you been sick?" I took two lessons from this interaction: (1) I didn't need to get to know Mary any better, and (2) I needed to cut myself some slack and realize I was doing the best I could. Do the best you can.

Summary

There is a lot of information in this chapter—about managing anxiety, uncertainty, your identity, and your self-presentation. That's a lot of management!

I hope you will find some comfort in the knowledge that you are not alone in experiencing anxiety and uncertainty. From there, perhaps there are one or two ideas you can use here to make you feel more in control of your experience. How each of us chooses to present ourselves to the world is deeply personal. Again, my hope is that you glean one or two strategies from my suggestions that might help you attain your self-presentation goals.

Notes

Notes

Chapter 4: Our Communities

In the midst of trying to wrap your own head around having breast cancer, you will also likely have to wrap your head around talking about it with other people. In this chapter, I focus on talking to people in family, social, and work networks. In chapter 5, I'll cover communicating with healthcare providers.

When I was first diagnosed, I wasn't particularly strategic about the way I disclosed my breast cancer. I was alone at home when I received my diagnosis. I called my husband, who was out of town. I also called my mom who lives across the country from me. She told my father and brother. I did not call anyone else in my family. I called a couple of friends the night of my diagnosis, but otherwise just let the news sink in. The day after my diagnosis, I emailed my closest friends to let them know, as well as to ask for their help identifying a surgeon in my area. A week later, I called my supervisor at work. Shortly thereafter, I emailed my department work colleagues because I was in search of someone to teach my classes for the year. I did not discuss my breast cancer on any social media platform. I emailed periodic updates to what became a large group of people.

I chose to disclose details to my closest family and friends, but even then, I did not tell them everything. It was just too much for me to share details about some of the most personal side effects I experienced. Even here, writing this book, I keep typing and deleting the hard to disclose details, concerned that my people will read this book and learn that I purposefully kept things from them because I did not want them to know about my toughest moments. Beyond the people closest to me, I did not disclose lots of detail unless people asked. I was willing to share about my disease because I wanted people to understand breast cancer better. I felt like this rabbit hole I had fallen down needed to be more public, more in the open. And I had an opportunity to facilitate that.

Talking to people about your cancer can be challenging. Cancer scares people, and it will likely scare people to learn that you have cancer. To help you navigate these conversations, I focus here on ways to think about your conversations and on strategies for specific kinds of interactions.

Telling People About Your Breast Cancer

Telling people you have cancer involves self-disclosure. Self-disclosure is an "interaction between at least two individuals where one intends to deliberately divulge something personal to another."[29] When we self-disclose, we move information, feelings, experiences, etc. from unknown to others to known to others. There is so much about us that other people can't know just by looking at us, including whether we have breast cancer. Surgery and radiation are invisible to most people around us, so those of us treated in this way have a broad range of things we can choose whether to self-disclose to others. Chemotherapy brings more visible signs of illness. Some of these signs can be managed to a degree (see chapter 3), but others indicate to people that we are undergoing treatment for cancer. Even with our cancer more obviously signaled to people, though, we have control over the details we disclose.

I realized early on that I had to think about how I was disclosing my cancer to people. A week after my diagnosis, I was at an open football practice at the University of Washington with my husband. As we were leaving, I saw our office administrator, someone I consider a friend. He greeted me and asked me how I was doing. I blurted out, "I have breast cancer." Sheesh. Not exactly my ideal self-disclosure. Here we were, at a fun event, seeing each other for the first time in a while, and I announced my cancer. In thinking about who I wanted to be through my experience, I realized that I wanted to be more purposeful when I told people I had cancer.

I soon began to think of my breast cancer self-disclosure in terms of 4 continua—about who, when, how much, and how to share information about my breast cancer. A continuum indicates degrees of difference between two extremes. For instance, black and white are two ends of a color continuum, with many shades of gray in between, many of which are indistinguishable from their adjacent shades. The 4 continua I describe here are interrelated, but I find it useful to look at them separately as a way to be more purposeful about a range of cancer conversations. These continua are not static.

Rather, they shift over time, across contexts, and across our communities. Most of us probably fall somewhere in the middle in general, but we may slide side to side on one or more of the continua as we engage some of the other dimensions of disclosure here.

The key to remember here is that this is about you. You get to decide who you tell, when you tell, how much you tell, and how you tell. There is so much we cannot control when we have breast cancer. It's totally reasonable to control the information about your cancer, about your story.

Who to Tell

No one ———————————————— Everyone

"Everyone" and "no one" are two ends of a continuum with lots of variations in between. For instance, you may choose to tell a lot of people about your breast cancer but draw your line at strangers. Or you may choose to keep your cancer diagnosis and treatment more private, telling only those with whom you interact on a daily basis at home, at work, and in your community. Few of us choose either "everyone" or "no one," especially as we consider the other three continua.

It's your choice who to tell about your cancer. Nonverbally, I pretty much announced to the world that I had cancer because I was bald. Even when my hair started to grow back and I thought I looked more like myself, people could tell that I had cancer. The clerk at the Department of Motor Vehicles took one look at me when I went to get my new license photo (3 months late because I forgot—thank you, chemo brain!), waived the late fees, and told me I could come back to get a new photo later. I didn't explicitly tell him that I had cancer, but he could tell, in part because he also had cancer.

You may choose to tell virtually no one. It's difficult, but not impossible, to keep your illness from your partner, family, and/or housemates. However, beyond those people with whom you are in closest contact, it can be pretty simple to keep your breast cancer private, especially if you have no outward signs of cancer or treatment. I know several women who told virtually no one that they had breast cancer.

When to Tell

Never ——————————————————— Immediately

The anchors of this continuum involve the timing of our disclosure. On one end, you never disclose your breast cancer. On the other end, you share your experience as it happens. Again, this is connected to the other continua. If, for instance, you think about who you tell, you may tell some people immediately (e.g., your partner or family) and you may never tell some people (e.g., people you meet after your treatment is over).

Odds are you will fall somewhere in between the continuum extremes. I told my husband information immediately but otherwise waited until I had a chance to process things myself before telling people. I told my Facebook friends only after I was done with all of my active treatments, nine months after my initial diagnosis. At that point, I posted this status update:

> *256 days ago, I learned I had early-stage breast cancer. Today, I finished my radiation treatment (after surgery and chemotherapy). I've spent more time on FB in the past months than usual, watching your lives unfold and occasionally chiming in. Thanks for sharing, and by doing so, keeping me distracted and sane. Oh, and if you're a woman over 40, get a mammogram, ok?*
>
> *Love,*
> *Lisa*

And this leads to the third continuum—how much to tell.

How Much to Tell

Nothing ——————————————————— Everything

Most of the details of our cancer are invisible to people. We get to decide how much to share. Some of us choose to share nothing that is not immediately obvious from the way we look. Others choose to share every detail of our cancer diagnosis, treatment, prognosis, thoughts, and feelings. As with the other continua, most of us likely fall somewhere in the middle, and we will slide to different points across time, people, and contexts.

At the beginning of my experience, I had very little information myself, only that I had breast cancer, so I shared all of that information with the people I chose to tell. Over time, I had an overwhelming amount of information about my tumor biology, my prognosis, my treatment, and my recovery process. I also had lots of feelings and thoughts about my cancer and life. I chose to disclose less and less, relative to what I knew and felt. For instance, I ended up with neuropathy that caused my body to burn anytime I sweated, which was frequent because I had severe hot flashes. I didn't share that information, even though it was a significant part of my experience for some time.

How much you tell people will likely be closely connected to who those people are. I told my closest people more than I told those I don't know well, but I also tended to try to protect people I cared about from knowing some of the most difficult things I experienced. As with other aspects of your story, you get to decide how much detail to share.

How to Tell

Privately ——————————————— Publicly

This continuum focuses on whether you use a relatively private form of communication or a relatively public one. There are many options when it comes to how to share information with people. You can talk face-to-face, on the phone, use email, create a page on a healthcare site like CaringBridge, post on your social media accounts, write a personal blog, and myriad others. These modes of communication vary in terms of their relative privacy. Face-to-face communication, for example, is private, whereas a personal blog is more public, unless it is password protected. In the middle are targeted emails to specific people and password-protected health update sites. It's important to remember, though, that emails can be forwarded and that information from password-protected sites can be shared with other people. You won't have complete control over whether your information is shared beyond the people you tell directly. It can be useful to think about how easily shareable the information you share is. There also may be situations in which you want your information shared by others, so that you don't have to tell people directly. This is helpful to bear in mind as you communicate with others.

Talking About Your Breast Cancer

You get to decide whether, to whom, when, and how you disclose your disease to people. There is no right mix of whether, to whom, when, and how to talk about your cancer. I communicated about my breast cancer to my family, close friends, acquaintances, close colleagues, general colleagues, and relative strangers. Although I tended to hang out at consistent areas of the four continua, I slid along each as the group changed and over the course of my experience. In general, I was pretty open about my disease. I shared details of my diagnosis and treatment plan with anyone who was interested because, as I mentioned earlier, I felt as though I was educating people about breast cancer. I generally told people when they asked, but sometimes that meant immediately and sometimes that meant after everything was over. And I told people in relatively private ways, knowing that the information could be shared.

I hope the continua provide a means to think through some options. Here are some examples of the changing nature of my breast cancer self-disclosures that may help you think strategically about your own self-disclosure. My examples are essentially snapshots of a moment in time during an experience that was actually quite fluid. Clearly, there are lots of shades of gray between any two snapshots. You'll notice that each of my examples includes 3 of the 4 continua. That's because each example makes one of the continua redundant. The first example is about what I did when I first had breast cancer. In other words, it's what I did "immediately" upon hearing I had cancer, making the "when to tell" continuum redundant.

When I first learned I had breast cancer, here's how my self-disclosure looked.

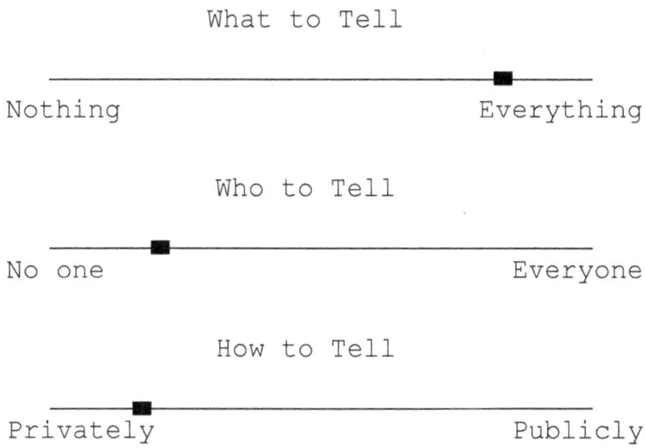

In the beginning, I wanted tight control over who knew about my cancer. I didn't have much information to share, so I shared it all. All I really knew in the beginning was that I had breast cancer. I shared the information privately, either by phone, text, or email. I didn't tell anyone immediately face-to-face, including my husband who was out of town.

When my treatment ended, things looked very different. Again, I'm excluding the "when to tell" continuum because this is how my communication looked "immediately" post-treatment.

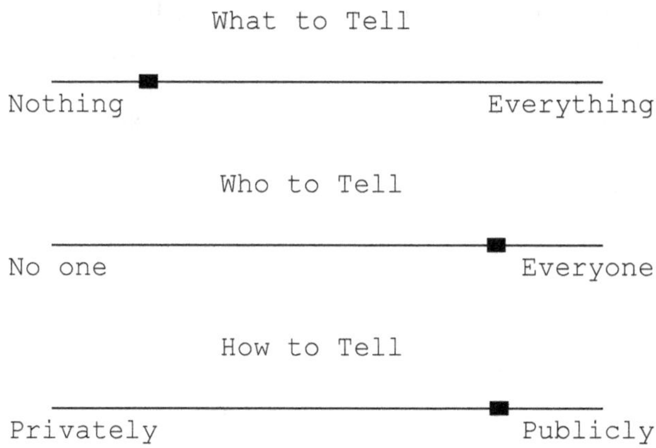

On my first day post-treatment, I disclosed my breast cancer on Facebook. I essentially told everyone I knew, but I told them very little. I mentioned my treatment but did not provide details. It was not a lot more information than I had myself at the very beginning of my experience, but it accounted for a very small amount of the information I had by the time my treatment was over.

In addition to shifting over time, my self-disclosure shifted from group to group. In the following 2 examples, I exclude the "who to tell" continuum because my examples are about who I actually told. With family and close friends, my continua mostly looked like this:

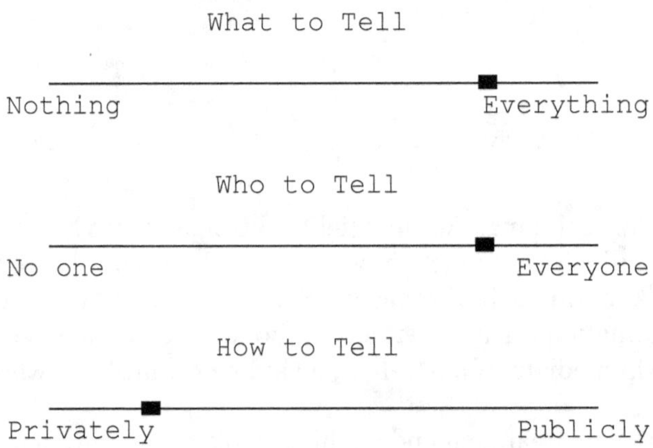

I tended to tell my family and close friends almost everything about my disease and treatment. I spared them some details, but I felt they could handle and help me through the hard things. This was a small group, but it also grew over time to include people who stepped toward me when I was sick, but who I wasn't close to before. I shared with individual people in either face-to-face conversations or via phone. I also shared with this entire group relatively privately, via occasional emails.

With acquaintances, my continua generally looked like this:

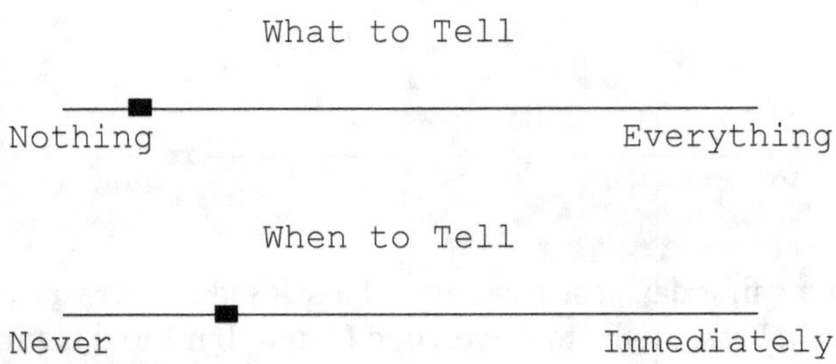

How to Tell

Privately ——■—————————— Publicly

I shared very little with acquaintances. I allowed long lapses between when something happened and when I told people. I tended to share the basics with acquaintances or near-strangers. I would tell people I had breast cancer but only provide few details. I also only told these people once I was comfortable with the information.

As you think about sharing information about your breast cancer, realize that you don't need to tell everyone yourself. You can rely on others to share your news. For instance, I asked some friends to let other friends know. And I relied on my parents and brother to let everyone in my extended family know about my diagnosis and treatment. It's even useful for some of the people in your inner circle to be able to tell people further out from you about your illness. It allows them to make some connections to people who can support them. Although I explicitly asked close friends and immediate family to tell others, I also learned that people at my work spread the word to people who cared about me, but who were not in my immediate work group. This was helpful, especially as I got further into treatment and looked less like my usual self at work. I didn't have to explain my situation because people already knew. Depending on your own needs, you may choose to enlist some close people to share your news for you. One benefit of this, which was important to me, was that it allows people to have their emotional responses to your diagnosis, treatment, and prognosis away from you, and then to connect with you later.

Be gentle with yourself as you deal with people's responses to what you tell them about your cancer. We all need to deal with other people's responses to our self-disclosures about our cancer, from the time we tell people we have cancer through treatment and beyond. One of the main reasons I didn't use Facebook to talk about my illness until it was over was that I didn't want to have to respond to people's responses. I conserved my energy for other things. Clinical psychologist Susan Silk and arbitrator/mediator Barry Goldman's Ring Theory is a useful model for thinking through communication with our people during our breast cancer experience, and for understanding what is appropriate for our people to communicate to us.[30]

Ring theory represents your social network and support structure as a set of concentric circles, with you in the middle and the circles around you representing people ranging from close to you to distant from you. People close to you, like your family, occupy a circle closely surrounding you. Other circles include close friends, acquaintances, work colleagues, and strangers. Who occupies each circle depends on you. Who are you closest to? Who is more distant? With this visual representation in place, the theory suggests that "support" should be expressed from people on the outer circles to people in the inner circles; conversely, people can only "vent" from the inner circles out.

Let me give you a couple of concrete examples. You, as the person in the center of the concentric circles can vent about your cancer to anyone in the outer circles. And any of those people can offer you support. Your acquaintances, however, can only vent about how they feel about your cancer to people on the periphery of the concentric circles and can only expect support from those same people. A close family member can vent to and expect support from anyone in your social network except you (because you are closer to the center of the concentric circles).

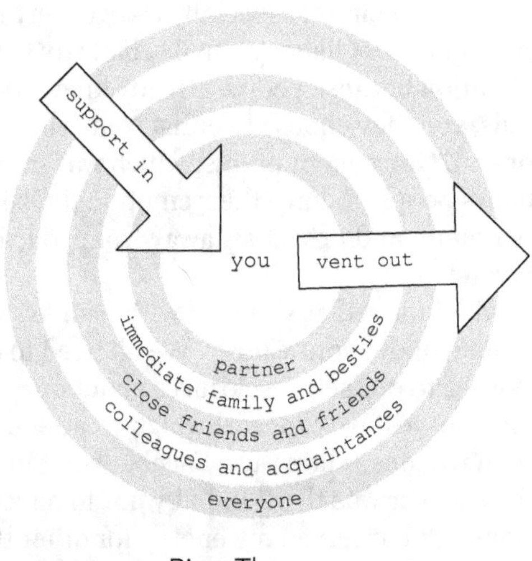

Ring Theory

People may respond to you in ways that are more about them than about you. They may cry, offer advice, tell stories, disagree with your treatment decisions, or say things you consider inappropriate.

It's okay to tell them that you don't want to talk to them about their feelings about your disease. As I mentioned earlier, one of the most difficult responses I dealt with was people telling me I was strong. I didn't feel strong and I told them so.

With people you care about, you will care about how they feel about your cancer. I found myself taking care of people sometimes. In response to one of my email updates, a friend remarked that my note functioned to assuage her and others' fears and worries, and that I didn't need to be doing that. She was right, but I wasn't even aware that I was taking care of others until she pointed it out.

Here are some examples of things I actually said to people who responded to me in ways that weren't helpful to me:

- Emotional responses of others (e.g., tears, worry, anger):

  I appreciate that you care so much.

  Thank you, but I can't be your emotional support right now. I have a lot on my plate.

- Unsolicited treatment advice:

  I really trust my doctors.

  Thank you, but I feel good about my plan.

- Unwanted stories:

  I'm glad your friend survived.

  Every breast cancer is really different.

  I don't really want to hear about people dying right now.

- Inappropriate comments:

  That's not really helpful to me right now.

  Please stop talking about that. I'm not on the same page.

It's not always easy to tell people you care about that you can't care *for* them when it comes to your cancer. But you are the most important character in your breast cancer story. Take care of yourself. And offer your friends and family the venting/supporting model to help explain your needs. As one of my doctors said to me, "Put your own oxygen mask on first."

Communicating Your Needs

Remember, again, that your needs are the most important part of the conversations you have with other people. From the very beginning of my experience, I was clear about my own needs when communicating with friends and family. When I disclosed my diagnosis via email, I told people it was because I was not ready to talk, but that I needed help getting a plan in place. I asked for the kind of help I needed—recommendations for doctors, companions for chemotherapy, someone to sit with me after surgery so my husband could work, someone to talk to, book recommendations, movie recommendations, etc.

Sometimes, people offered me things that I did not need or want and telling them that was difficult. The hardest one was that my mother wanted to come see me as soon as possible after my diagnosis. She lives across the country from me, so that meant that she would be staying in my home for an extended period of time. I was overwhelmed and I needed time and space to get my head around what was happening to me. Ultimately, after a conversation about what would work best for me, she and my father came to see me mid-way through my chemotherapy. By then, I knew more what to expect during my treatment and my parents were able to be incredibly helpful when I needed it most.

Lots of people wanted to get together during this time, but I just didn't have the energy to see people. I think that my friends would have been okay with a low energy version of me, but I wasn't. I didn't want to hang out with people when I wasn't feeling well. Toward the end of my chemotherapy treatments, I felt so sick that I could not even hold a phone conversation with my closest friends. I knew that people were just trying to be helpful and kind, and I felt bad about refusing visits, meals, etc. But refuse I did. I hope people understood.

Telling Your Employer

If you are employed, you will likely need to inform your

workplace of your cancer diagnosis. However, what you need to disclose to whom will vary depending on where you work. You do have workplace rights, and it is important that you know what those are (cancerandcareers.org/en/at-work/legal-and-financial/cancer-and-the-ada-fmla).

Talk to Human Resources (HR), if your place of employment has an HR office. In most situations, you will not be the first person in your workplace to have had cancer. If you are unable to get the answers you need from your workplace, cancerandcareers.org is a good place to look for information and guidance. HR should be able to guide you through the process of requesting workplace accommodations or leave during and after your treatment.

I had a very positive experience at my workplace, a large public university. The human resources people made it clear to me that I had rights regarding leave from work for treatment and that they would help me navigate the system. As a faculty member at my institution, I had no sick days. I was, however, entitled to long-term illness leave regulated by the Family and Medical Leave Act (FMLA). The staff also made it clear that my leave was an HR issue, and that I did not need to tell any of my coworkers or my department chair what was going on with my health. Luckily, I was able to use FMLA throughout my entire treatment and beginning recovery.

Every workplace is different. You know the atmosphere of your workplace. Trust yourself and your choices around sharing your diagnosis, treatment, and prognosis.

Communicating with Children

Tell children what they need to know. I don't have children, so I can't offer you my own experience of talking to them. I have lots of friends with breast cancer who have children, though, and I've witnessed how they interact with them about their breast cancer. One close friend, who was diagnosed when her daughter was 22 months old, wanted to make sure that she helped her daughter understand the parts of her illness and treatment that would be most visible to her. She explained to her daughter that she was going to have some medicine that would make her more tired than usual and would cause her to lose her hair. When it came time for the mastectomy, she explained that the doctors would take away the cancerous parts that were making her sick. All along, she reassured her daughter that her doctors were taking good care of her. I recently asked her if she had advice I could offer in this book. Her response was, "It depends" on your cancer and your child—who she is, how she thinks about her world, how old she is, what other experiences she's had with cancer.

One study revealed that women with breast cancer and their male partners sometimes try to protect children by not talking with them about their mother's cancer. However, this strategy can backfire and cause both the children and the parents increased stress when children fill in the blanks on their own and need parents to then correct the children's information.[31]

Experts on talking to children about breast cancer suggest that you consider age and development when you tell them about your cancer.[32] Tell minor children what they need to know in simple, direct language. For instance, young children likely need to know that you're sick and whether their daily lives will be affected. Adolescents can handle more information and involvement in your experience, but may also have concerns you'll need to address about how your cancer will affect them. Adult children can be treated like any other adult, except for the fact that you are their mother with a serious illness. Adult children may also be concerned about their own cancer risk. Whether, how much, and when you tell your children about your breast cancer is, again, up to you. But experts tend to advise that the children's age and development guide the type and amount of information you share.

Here are a few online sites that provide helpful, specific suggestions about how to talk with your children:

- Breast Cancer Now: breastcancernow.org/about-breast-cancer/primary-breast-cancer/talking-with-children-about-breast-cancer
- Komen: komen.org/wp-content/uploads/Talking-with-your-Children.pdf
- Living Beyond Breast Cancer: lbbc.org/about-breast-cancer/familyrelationships/parenting/talking-children-about-breast-cancer
- Living Beyond Breast Cancer: lbbc.org/wp-content/uploads/2022/07/Reading-for-Reassurance-Discussion-Guide-2022-ages-4-7-digital.pdf

Summary

Choosing how to talk about your cancer is all about weaving your breast cancer experience into your larger life story. Part of that, for me, was figuring out how other people fit into my story. Who were the other characters? I thought about my family and close friends as my "raggedy love army," a term I borrowed from author Anne Lamott. On August 12, 2014, Lamott reflected about Robin Williams' death on her public Facebook page. In her anguish, she wished for something more than the helpers we turn to when things in life are hard, but she also recognized that our own personal raggedy love armies of helpers get us through the worst of our life, just as we help them through the worst of their lives. These were the people I counted on to hold me up, just as they could count on me to hold them up. Not everyone I encountered was part of this group, but these people became a key part of my story. Toward the end of my treatment, I sent my raggedy love army this message:

> *I know I've said it before, but I really don't think I can say it enough. Thank you for keeping me going. I talk to you in my head (I know it's weird, but I do!); I feel your love; and I lean on you when I just don't think I can take another day of treatment. You've made my life easier.*
>
> *Love,*
> *Lisa*

My story continues to develop, and my updates to my raggedy love army have become less and less frequent. As you make choices about your own cancer conversations, you will also craft the storyline and characters of the chapter that includes your breast cancer.

Notes

Notes

Notes

Chapter 5: Our Healthcare Network

Cancer and Communication

A group of researchers from M.D. Anderson Cancer Center asserted that "communication is the cornerstone of comprehensive cancer care."[33] Communication with our group of healthcare providers is an important part of breast cancer treatment, recovery, and survival. Frankly, I was surprised by how many people were involved with my care and all of the communication my care required.

Communication affects health in several ways. Specifically, communication with our healthcare providers affects our knowledge of our health, our sense of agency or control, and the quality of our treatment decisions.[34] Even though all of my healthcare providers were in contact with each other to some degree, I was the common thread linking them together and I tried to be proactive in ensuring they were all up to date on what was going on with me.

I found managing the logistics of appointments challenging. "Challenging" became "overwhelming" when I added in trying to manage my relationships and identity during all of my healthcare provider interactions. All communication involves both content and relational messages. Content messages involve the exchange of information. Relational messages implicitly or explicitly signal our connections to the people with whom we're interacting. These relational messages are part of our identity. In a conversation with your surgeon, for example, you may ask questions about your surgical options, and in the way you ask, you may also convey to the surgeon whether you are confident in her abilities, relying on her to make decisions for you, and/or demonstrate your knowledge of your options.

At one point, as I was sobbing in my cancer psychiatrist's office, she said, "Maybe you should stop trying to be the perfect cancer patient." Even though I studied and taught communication for a living, I found myself stuck at times, not knowing how to talk to the people who were involved with my care. I wanted them to like me and sometimes that overrode my ability to ask for help from the very people who could see me through some of my toughest moments.

There are thousands of research articles on physician-patient communication and breast cancer. Much of this research focuses on helping providers make sure patients are involved in their care, get the care they need/want, and feel supported along the way. This is a good thing to remember: Healthcare providers know that communication matters and they want to help you get what you need. Styles differ, of course, so part of choosing your providers is finding people whose style works for you. Not nearly as many research articles provide how-to communication guidance for patients. What does exist demonstrates that communication makes a difference in patients' quality of care and quality of outcomes.[35]

Much of the research on patient communication focuses on treatment decision conversations with surgeons and medical oncologists, which makes sense because these are consequential moments in the breast cancer experience. Unfortunately, "doctors tend to overestimate their ability in communication"[36] so we can't count on them to take full responsibility for our interactions, as much as they might be doing their best. Physicians and patients also have some important differences in what they consider to be helpful and unhelpful provider communication, especially around patient sexual health. Sexual health can be a sensitive topic that many patients noted could be addressed more directly, comprehensively, and openly by their physicians.[37] This all means that you have some opportunities to take charge of your interactions with your healthcare providers. Being strategic about your communication can help maximize the positive outcomes of your healthcare interactions.

I could not always implement what I knew intellectually I needed to do. In this chapter, I will demystify the various healthcare communication encounters you're apt to experience, and I'll offer some strategies for managing the communication in these interactions. Some basic communication concepts can come in handy. My hope is to empower you to be as proactive in your care as you'd like to be. After my cancer psychiatrist's comment about being the perfect cancer patient, I embraced imperfection in every aspect of my communication during my cancer experience. I hope you do too.

Patient-Focused Research on Patient-Provider Communication

My experience with breast cancer recast my thinking of cancer treatment as something strictly scientific to something that is part science and part art. As mentioned above, most of the communication research on cancer and communication focuses on how healthcare providers can better communicate with their patients. This makes sense because of the impact high quality communication from healthcare providers can have on many people. However, this book is about you and about providing you with tools to advocate for yourself during your breast cancer experience.

Much of the research on patient communication with providers revolves around two themes: information seeking and treatment decision-making. These two themes dominated much of my healthcare experience. Here, I explain what the research tells us about these two areas and then transition to some strategies for communicating with different healthcare providers and in specific cancer-related communication contexts.

The research themes answer two important, related questions that you'll face: How do I get the information I need and want, and how do I make decisions about my treatment? The underlying assumptions of these research threads is that patient-centered communication and patient involvement in treatment decisions can have positive influences on patient satisfaction with their treatment decisions,[38] health outcomes,[39] and anxiety.[40] The research identifies some correlations between communication and patients' experiences. For example, the more surgeons discuss possible outcomes with women, the more satisfied women report being with their medical treatment and health outcomes, regardless of their ultimate surgery choice.[41] Many studies investigate the use of communication interventions that promote patient question asking,[42] but some of these studies don't detail how the timing of patients' questions might impact their satisfaction. For example, at presurgical consultations, when patients asked questions that were not in response to a surgeon asking for questions, they tended to be less satisfied with their treatment plan and their surgeon, and less likely to comply with their treatment plan.[43] And even though there is an emphasis on involving patients in treatment decision-making, the most important decision-making factor in patient satisfaction and improvement in health outcomes is whether their actual involvement in decision-making aligns with their desired involvement.[44] This factor dovetails well with my goal for you in this book—to decide what works for you. The most important part of communicating with your care team is to figure out how you want to be involved in decision-making around your care and then to enact a plan to make that happen.

Healthcare providers encourage patients to ask questions. At my first appointment with my surgeon, I received a binder of materials to read, including encouragement to ask questions. It even included a list of some great example questions to get me started. I exhausted the list of about 50 questions pretty quickly, especially considering that I had more than 100 appointments during my 9 months of active treatment. (If you want a full list of the questions I asked, see chapter 3.)

The current approach to decision-making prioritizes patient-centered care, actively involving patients in decision-making.[45] This approach is based in Self-Determination Theory, which proposes that our "experienced quality of life is largely a matter of the degree to which three basic psychological needs for autonomy, competence and relatedness are met."[46] What this means is that if you feel like you have some personal control over your care (autonomy), you are able to navigate the various contexts of your care (competence), and you feel connected to those helping you (relatedness), you'll also feel like you're experiencing a higher quality of life. Finding care providers that work with your preferred communication style is a great first step in optimizing your care and meeting your needs for autonomy, competence, and relatedness.

Demographics, in particular patient race, also play a role in how we experience our healthcare. As I noted in the beginning of this book, I am a White, straight, married, child-free woman, so I can only offer my own experience from my own demographic perspective. However, I know from my reading that women of color in particular have different breast cancer communication experiences than White women. For example, African American and Latina women have reported more regret and less decision quality than White women.[47] Beyond differences in our perceptions, which are relatively subjective, researchers have observed age, race, education, and income differences in how doctors and patients communicate, with the most consistent difference being in patient race. In one study, younger, White, and more highly-educated people asked more questions and provided more biomedical information than others to their physicians; likewise, physicians tended to provide more biomedical information and connect more relationally with these patients than others. Physicians also tended to ask more questions of non-white, less educated, and low-income patients.[48] In another study of how cancer-care providers talk with their African American and Latina patients, researchers found that providers recognized differences in their patients' cultural beliefs and demographics, but tended to provide cancer information and education in the same way across all patients.[49] Exactly how demographic categories influence our care is not yet clearly understood, as other research has found that race/ethnicity didn't specifically align with differences in patient quality of life.[50]

So, what can we take away from this somewhat contradictory research? I highlight demographic categories here because disparities in healthcare persist, even if we don't completely understand the mechanisms or solutions. While there is a lot of research focused on improving practitioners' communication with their patients of color, I did not find any research that provided guidance on how people of color can empower themselves to shape the conversations with their care providers. We enter our breast cancer experience with our own set of demographic characteristics. Recognizing when, where, and how demographics are consequential in our own care is another opportunity to empower ourselves to manage our healthcare interactions. In the strategies section below, I provide some links to online resources that do provide breast cancer information specific to women of color.

Healthcare Characters

Cancer care involves many providers. I never expected my life story to include a cast of cancer healthcare characters. You probably didn't either. But a cast of healthcare providers comes with the breast cancer territory. At a minimum, breast cancer treatment involves a breast surgeon and a medical oncologist (and their staffs). Depending on treatment, there may also be a radiation oncologist, radiation technologists, radiation nurses, chemotherapy infusion nurses, lab technicians, pathologists, physical therapists, an onco-physiatrist, a plastic surgeon, a massage therapist, a naturopath, an acupuncturist, and a psychiatrist or social worker.

Each of these people plays a different role in your care, with the common goal of helping you. A *breast surgeon*, usually the first healthcare provider you see after diagnosis, performs breast surgery to remove as much cancer as possible. She may also remove lymph nodes to assess whether your cancer has spread beyond the breast. *Medical oncologists* treat breast cancer with chemotherapy and other drugs (such as endocrine therapies). *Radiation oncologists* plan radiation treatments, including target areas, dose strength, and duration. *Radiation technologists* administer radiation treatments. *Radiation nurses* guide you through the radiation process and serve as a liaison between the radiation technologists and radiation oncologists. *Chemotherapy infusion nurses* administer chemotherapy medications and monitor you through the infusion process. *Lab technicians* perform regular blood work (especially before chemotherapy). *Pathologists* analyze biopsies and tumor samples. *Physical therapists* help support your fitness plan, address any treatment-caused physical conditions, including lymphoma, and create an at-home plan with you. *Onco-physiatrists* create a fitness plan for you to optimize health during treatment. *Plastic surgeons* reconstruct breasts (according to your desired outcome) after mastectomies and revise surgery scars. *Massage therapists* treat muscle and tissue problems that result from stress and treatment. *Naturopaths* provide complementary treatments to support your body through surgery, chemotherapy, and radiation. *Acupuncturists* help alleviate treatment side-effects. *Psychiatrists, psychologists,* or *social workers* help you manage emotional, relational, and social effects of breast cancer. In addition to these central characters, your healthcare team will include schedulers, receptionists, and nurses who support both your healthcare provider and you as you progress through treatment.

Women of Color

Women of color face communication challenges in cancer-care contexts. The following online resources provide information and support specific to how women of color experience breast cancer. They do not provide as much concrete communication advice as I would like to see, but there is not a lot of concrete communication advice in general for how women can improve their communication with their cancer-care providers (hence, this book!). My hope is that the resources here can help you connect to communities of people who understand your lived experience.

- For the Breast of Us is an organization focused on empowering women of color through education, advocacy, and community. breastofus.com/for-the-breast-of-us-empowering-women-of-color-through-advocacy-community-and-education

- The Breast Cancer Research Foundation website includes discussions of disparities in breast cancer treatment and outcomes for African American, AAPI, Native, and Hispanic and Latina women. www.bcrf.org/about-breast-cancer/breast-cancer-racial-disparities
- African American Breast Cancer Alliance provides hope, awareness, education, emotional and social support to breast cancer survivors, their family members and the community. aabcainc.org/black-women-and-breast-cancer
- Sisters is a national African American breast cancer survivorship organization that provides resources and connections for African American women. www.sistersnetworkinc.org

Healthcare Provider Communication Strategies

The research coupled with my personal experience helped me create a list of strategies I wish I had when I was in active treatment.

Take advantage of any communication and decision aids offered by your healthcare provider or healthcare center.
Because communication is such a central part of the breast cancer medical experience, there are resources available to help you maximize your communication with your healthcare providers. These aids range from lists of questions (like the one I received at my first surgical appointment), to communication coaching, to question prompts before each appointment, to online support systems, to aids designed specifically to help you make treatment decisions. Communication and decision aids have been shown to help us attain better quality of life,[51] and increase our self-efficacy while reducing our anxiety.[52] You are not the first person to wonder how to be in control in the foreign land of cancer. If your healthcare provider does not provide communication and decision aids, you can look online for some assistance by searching for "question prompt lists for breast cancer" or use the list of questions I provided in chapter 3 as a resource.

You can ask your healthcare providers anything.
There is no silly question. Ask about what you want to know. I tended to freeze somewhat at my appointments. Even now, I have questions before I get to my appointment, but I forget them if I don't write them down. I kept a notebook with questions and answers for every appointment to help me remember what questions to ask and what responses I got. I brought my husband with me to most major appointments. He made sure I asked the questions in my book and he recorded the answers. You can also record your appointments on a smartphone. As a matter of fact, the healthcare team for my second opinion recorded the appointment for future reference.

Healthcare Provider Communication Strategies (Continued)

Decide how much information you want.
I mentioned in chapter 3 that we all differ in the amount of information we want or need about our breast cancer. We differ in the number of questions we ask and the amount of information we seek. However, research has found that most women want as much information as possible about their breast cancer.[53] Because I function better with more information, I asked lots of questions. You should ask the kind and number of questions you need to satisfy your own level of desired information.

I found the limits of my own need for information shortly after I completed active treatment. I asked my medical oncologist what I should say to people about my cancer—was I cured? in remission? I study language so this was important to me. He said that the medical community doesn't generally use the words "cure" or "remission" for breast cancer, but that I could say that I had completed initial treatment for my breast cancer and that I was currently free of clinically detectable disease. When I told him that that wasn't exactly heartwarming, he smiled wryly and said, "You asked."

Ask your questions in the appropriate form.
Once you know what information you want, the next step is to figure out how to ask questions. How you ask a question can affect the answer you get. To be clear, it won't change the accuracy of the information you get in the answer, but it might change how much information you get or whether you get an answer to the question you hoped to ask.

Questions can be open or closed. Open questions are broad, information-seeking questions that allow the respondent to provide a range of responses. These are who, what, where, why, how questions. Closed questions ask for more specific information and limit the kinds of responses a person can give. These are often yes/no or limited option response questions. Thinking strategically about how you ask questions can help ensure that you get the information you seek.

Healthcare Provider Communication Strategies (Continued)

You may, for instance, be wondering about treatment options. You can ask very open-ended questions like, "What treatment do you think I will need?" which allows the healthcare provider free rein in responding. You also might ask a more closed question like, "Will I need chemotherapy?" This question focuses on a specific topic and directly requests a yes, no, maybe response. At different points in your experience, you will likely need different kinds of information. Asking a question in a form that fits the information you want can facilitate the interaction between you and your healthcare provider.

Similarly, it can be useful to think of primary questions and follow-up questions. A primary question can be either open or closed, but it gets at the crux of the issue you want addressed. Depending on the answer you receive, you may have follow-up questions. So, for instance, with the primary question, "Will I need chemotherapy?" I would have many follow up questions if I received a "yes" response: "What drugs?" "How long will the treatment last?" "What are the side effects of the medications?" "Will I be able to work during the treatment?" It can be helpful to write your questions out in advance of each appointment so they are structured to get you the information you desire.

Be explicit with your healthcare providers about how involved you want to be in decision-making. As with our desire for the amount of information we want, we can think about the desire to be involved in decision-making as a continuum. On one end are those of us who want to be deeply involved in making decisions; on the other end are those of us who choose a set of healthcare providers we trust and want the professionals to identify the best course of action. It is useful to figure out where you fall on this decision-making continuum and to let your healthcare providers know. There is no right or wrong way to approach this process.

I had choices to make regarding my treatment. I needed surgery, but I could either have a lumpectomy or mastectomy. The surgeon was fine with whichever choice I made, although she provided me

Healthcare Provider Communication Strategies (Continued)

with information to help me make the decision. There were also conflicting opinions on whether I needed chemotherapy. And if I decided to go ahead with chemotherapy, I had choices between different cocktails and whether to join a clinical trial. My husband, my medical oncologist, and I gathered information, talked through research studies, and all arrived at the same conclusion independently—that I should have chemo, but could opt for the less toxic cocktail. I also decided to participate in the clinical trial. Even so, the doctor made it clear that this was all my decision, that he would only order the chemotherapy with my go ahead.

I needed to be active in the decisions around my treatment. It was important to me. Yet I was acutely aware that I was not qualified to be making these decisions on my own. Working collaboratively with my doctors worked for me. The same may be true for you. Or you may prefer to have your physicians decide your treatment plans for you. Regardless of your preference for your own level of involvement in decision-making, you'll likely feel better about your treatment decisions if your physician communicates with you in a way that acknowledges your autonomy.[54]

Communication Contexts of Treatment

Cancer treatment involves managing communication in many new healthcare contexts. Each of these new contexts calls for new communication strategies. Here, I describe the verbal and nonverbal aspects of various treatment contexts and then offer some ideas for how to communicate in each. My goal is to give you a sense of what to expect in each context in order to decrease your uncertainty and increase your self-efficacy.

Chemotherapy

Unless you have accompanied someone else to chemotherapy, you probably don't have much, if any, experience in a chemotherapy infusion area. The chemotherapy infusion areas vary from facility to facility. I always had a somewhat private space, separated from other people by a curtain. Other people I know had their infusions in large rooms with all of the chairs in a big circle. The physical setting enables and constrains interactions with other patients, with infusion nurses, and with a companion.

Before my first chemotherapy treatment, my psychiatrist warned me that the waiting room was like an airport waiting area when a flight is delayed. Everyone is tense and waiting, and no one wants to be there. She suggested that I think about how I wanted to interact with other people in that setting, and to be strategic about the nonverbal and verbal cues I transmitted to signal my desire to those around me. Once I was in the infusion area itself, the nurses were friendly, professional, and compassionate, and I had minimal contact with other patients.

Radiation Treatment

The radiation waiting room was very different than the chemotherapy waiting room for me. Where the chemotherapy waiting room felt like a tense airport boarding area, the radiation treatment waiting room seemed more like an old-time jail (a friendly jail, but a jail nonetheless).

When I arrived for my first radiation treatment, I felt like an outsider. People in the waiting area knew each other and talked with each other. One of the most common questions I heard asked was (seriously!), "What are you in for?" Another was, "How many days do you have?" These questions made me think of old western movies when the inmates in the sheriff's office discuss their various crimes. Also, unlike chemotherapy waiting areas, radiation waiting areas are filled with people who have treatment every day at the same time for weeks. You tend to see the same people over and over again.

During one of the conversations I had in the radiation waiting room, a man asked me how many treatments I had to do. I told him 35. He responded that that was the highest number he had heard from anyone yet. He went on to tell me that he was 87 years-old and that he was having radiation to treat a cancer that his doctor told him wouldn't kill him. He asked me—a 47-year-old woman with a cancer that would kill me if left untreated—whether I thought the treatment was all worth it. I told him yes. And I avoided him in the waiting room from that point on.

The radiation oncologist constructs a treatment plan; she or her nurse is the patient's main point of contact. The radiation technologists administer the treatment. I had at least five different radiation technologists. Each one was kind, warm, and highly competent. Given my anxiety level about the treatment, these people made all the difference in the world to me. Early on, I told them that radiation was a breeze compared to chemotherapy. They exchanged a look and told me I'd probably feel different in a couple of weeks. They were right. It got harder. I experienced burning, blistering, and intense fatigue. I appreciated their honesty and knowing they were prepared for me to feel less well as my treatment progressed.

Radiation treatments are not long, but they can be uncomfortable because you have to stay very still. You will have a call button that the technologists expect you to use if you are having trouble. They will be in the next room, watching you on monitors and through a window.

One day, I had a very difficult radiation treatment. The Active Breathing Coordinator™ machine wasn't working properly so the technologists had to repeat images. I was uncomfortable, frustrated, and crying, but I had to stay as still as possible so that I wouldn't have to be repositioned, thus making the treatment even longer. Finally, we had to abandon the treatment for the day. I left the room in tears. As I passed the reception desk, the scheduler asked if I was okay. After I changed back into my clothes, I exited the dressing room to find the scheduler and the receptionist waiting for me with hugs and a glass of water. The scheduler asked if I wanted to talk to the radiation oncology nurse. I said I was okay, but saw the nurse walking toward me anyway. I talked to her for a while, cried quite a bit, and then left the radiation area. As I was walking through the lobby, the main floor greeter hugged me. A few minutes later, the radiation technologist called me on my cell phone to tell me that none of what happened was my fault and that he really hoped I would come back the following day to continue my treatments. He was sorry I felt so bad and said that he and his partner looked forward to seeing me every day. I did return the next day, accompanied by my husband for support.

Other Hospital Spaces

You will likely interact with other people at your care facility: Receptionists, pharmacists, security guards, and lab technicians. It's up to you how and how much you want to interact with the people around you. I found that talking to people who were not directly involved in my care helped me feel more normal. I liked saying hello to the receptionists and talking about local college sports with the security guard.

Summary

You will find yourself in new, unfamiliar settings as you work through your breast cancer diagnosis and treatment. It's easy to feel overwhelmed and lacking control. The healthcare providers you meet know that communication is an essential part of your diagnosis and treatment. Using the information in this chapter can hopefully help you be more purposeful in how you communicate with your healthcare providers and understand more fully the healthcare contexts of your treatment. If all else fails, remember that people are there to help you. The best advice I can give you is to ask for what you need.

General Chemotherapy Communication Strategies

Wear headphones and sit away from people if you don't want to talk to people in the waiting area.
Avoid eye contact with other people in the room. Respond minimally to people who ask you questions or greet you. This is not rude. This is self-preservation, if your choice is to limit your interaction with others.

Interact with people when you choose.
Smile, look at people, say hello, and sit close to people. If people respond in kind, then it's perfectly fine to chat. If people do any of the things listed above in number 1, it's probably best to find someone else to engage.

Decide whether you want to have a companion on your chemo days.
I had someone come with me every time. Some of them sat with me the whole time while others came and went throughout the day. As my chemotherapy treatments progressed, they became longer because I had some reactions to the medications that called for slower administration of them. The days were long and having company helped me.

The people who came with me played games with me, grabbed me water, brought me coffee, and talked with me. All of these things helped pass the time. They also worked on their laptops, watched me sleep, and went for walks around the neighborhood.

Decide what you want to do during your chemotherapy infusions regardless of whether you have a companion.
Other than communicating with the infusion nurses and my companion, I found chemotherapy to be a relatively communication-free place. To keep myself occupied, I had a chemotherapy bag that I brought to every appointment. It contained a blanket, snacks, books, magazines, candy, music, my phone, and my laptop. I also wrote all of my Christmas cards during one treatment. After all, I had time. As the treatments progressed and I became more fatigued, I also slept quite a bit. Although not communication advice, per se, these things helped me deal with the long quiet hours of my infusions.

Infusion Nurse Communication Strategies

Communicating with infusion nurses is extremely important. They are there to make sure your needs are met during the infusion. Two nurses will start your infusion to ensure that the correct medications and doses are given to the right person. There is a lot of quality control in chemotherapy infusions, and these are present to ensure your safety.

Ask any questions you have. They are there to help you.
Some example questions you might ask:

- Why do I get the medications separately instead of at the same time?
- How long will this infusion take?
- Is there anything I should be doing during treatment?
- How much water should I drink?
- Can I go use the bathroom with my IV or do you need to disconnect me first?
- Do you have any snacks?
- Can I have a blanket?

Tell the nurses if you experience any discomfort or pain.
The nurses will check in on you throughout your infusion, but don't wait to alert them if you don't feel well. You will have a call button that is meant to be used. Several times during my infusions, I called the nurses in to let them know that I was uncomfortable or that I had a concern about how I was feeling. They want to know what is going on with you. You are not bothering them. The more information they have about what you are experiencing, the more they can make your current and future infusions easier for you. If you are not comfortable letting the nurses know what is going on, be sure to bring a companion who can function as an advocate for you.

Radiation Treatment Communication Strategies

Decide whether you want to interact with people. Some people in the radiation waiting area were very chatty; others kept to themselves. Sometimes people's companions were chatty, too. I tended to want to interact some days and keep to myself other days, depending on how I was feeling physically and emotionally. On the days I wanted to interact, I sat close to other people, said hello, and smiled. On days I didn't want to interact, I often brought a book, sat further away from people, and said a quick hello at most.

Tell the radiation technologists if you are experiencing discomfort.

Notes

Notes

Notes

Chapter 6: Our Relationships

In some ways, cancer changed nothing for me. Even when I was my sickest, I was still myself with all of my good and bad points. In other ways, cancer changed everything, including my relationships with other people. Breast cancer impacts romantic relationships, family relationships, and friendships. Understandably, my healthcare providers were focused on saving my life (and I'm immensely grateful that they did). What they didn't or couldn't focus on at the time was what my life beyond cancer and its treatment looked like and how my life would change as a result of the experience.

We all experience individual turning points in our lives, those moments when our lives go from "before" to "after" (as I wrote about in chapter 3 about the shift from before diagnosis to after). In addition to these individual turning points, we all experience relational befores and afters.[55] These might be before or after a marriage, divorce, birth of a child, death of a child, or some other life change that redefines our relationships with significant others. Cancer catalyzes relational turning points in couples, in families, and in friendships. In this chapter, I provide an overview of some of the research on relationships and breast cancer, share some of my own experiences, and offer communication suggestions for weathering these changes.

Romantic and Family Relationships

A breast cancer diagnosis can affect the dynamics and balance in relationships with significant others. Relational issues are so central to the breast cancer experience that some researchers recommend studying "relational uncertainty" with "illness uncertainty."[56] Both women with breast cancer and our relational partners experience changes in our lives because of cancer.[57] These changes can be to our roles (e.g., family, medical support), emotions (e.g., increased depression or anxiety), priorities, and/or bodies.[58] Amidst these myriad changes, couples can become more intimate (defined by the article authors as "the perceived emotional closeness of the relationship") if they work together to not only deal with the cancer, but also to lead as normal a life as possible while acknowledging the ways that cancer impacts their identities and relationship.[59]

Relational partners are often our primary social support during our breast cancer experience. Couples' communication is important to understand, particularly how that communication contributes to or improves the psychological distress we experience. There is a lot of research on communication in couples where one partner has cancer, focusing especially on couples' openness and avoidance around cancer-related topics. One study found that women who talk about their cancer and cancer challenges with their partners are more likely to avoid blaming themselves for their cancer and more likely to seek support from others. All of these things contribute to a better psychological state.[60] The research, however, is varied. In fact, another study reviewed studies on couples' openness and avoidance and found that couples vary in their preferred communication amount and type.[61] So, while some research shows that being open about cancer-related topics is related to better psychological adjustment, it is important to remember that what works for one couple may not work for another.

Most of the communication research on relationships and breast cancer focuses on heterosexual couples. However, a recent study compared lesbian and heterosexual couples' communication during breast cancer treatment.[62] The authors found that lesbian couples talked more about caregiving and their partners' illness than did their heterosexual counterparts. This difference in the way lesbian and heterosexual partners communicated mirrored different male/female approaches to illness found in earlier research. The authors suggest that lesbian couples approached cancer as a shared experience, and the resulting communication could lead to better coping and less distress than heterosexual couples experienced.[63] Recognizing our own and our partners' communication preferences and patterns can help us make conscious choices about how we interact with each other during our breast cancer experience.

I so clearly remember the moment I discovered how my husband thought about my breast cancer in our relationship. He and I were driving away from the cancer center after my first appointment with my medical oncologist. The doctor had said that, given my relatively young age, he would likely recommend chemotherapy even if the cancer had not spread beyond my breast. I was shaken. I thanked my husband for coming with me. He paused and told me not to thank him. We were both taken aback. And then he said, "This is not happening just to you; it's happening to us." He was right. But I was used to being independent, and I could feel the balance of our relationship shifting in that moment. This shared view of our cancer remained throughout my treatment and long into my recovery.

My experience was not unique. Experiencing cancer not only changes how we as individuals think of ourselves, but also changes how we and our partners think about our relationship.[64] Couples tend to adapt more easily to the disease if they (1) take a couples approach to the cancer, (2) continue to seek ways to be a couple, (3) share similar ideas about cancer, and (4) are sensitive to each other's moods and emotions when choosing whether and what to communicate.[65]

The ways couples adapt to a breast cancer reality vary, just as the way couples function generally varies. My reading of the research on couples and communication revealed some of the usual biases in research. Most of the participants in the studies I cite here were White and heterosexual, with early-stage breast cancer. Clearly, we need more research on diverse populations, both in terms of communication and in terms of breast cancer interventions. What the research on couples does highlight is that there is not one right way to communicate with our partners. For instance, one study found that couples have an easier time talking about logistical and practical issues (e.g., healthcare providers) than potentially emotional ones (e.g., sexuality, fears of recurrence or death), and that the more couples avoid cancer-related topics, the more women experience anxiety, depression, and stress.[66] Another study found that women and their partners who avoid talking about what they consider inappropriate cancer-related topics feel satisfied in their relationships.[67] How we talk to our partners is only one factor influencing how we feel about our cancer experience; communication doesn't "cause" our feelings. When thinking about the social support relational partners provide to each other, it's important to remember that support is not a one-size-fits-all process. Instead, what we perceive as supportive, and therefore what makes us feel more satisfied in our relationships and less stressed, varies across couples and across the contexts in which couples interact.[68]

Dan and I had been married for 18 years when I was diagnosed. We'd been through a lot of life together. Breast cancer highlighted our strengths and weaknesses as individuals and a couple. One of the hallmarks of our relationship is that we are both very independent people. We spend a lot of time together, but we can also very happily function on our own. After my diagnosis, this shifted a bit. I was no longer able to be totally independent. I needed Dan in a way that I hadn't before. He was there.

My husband's independent streak became more pronounced. He said that taking care of me was his job. He refused help from other people, where I would have been more willing to accept it. That doesn't mean that we didn't have help; it's just that I was the person more likely to reach out to others for assistance or to say yes when it was offered. He didn't share a lot of how he was feeling with me, and I worried about him getting burned out. When I asked one of his friends to hang out with him to give him a break, he got angry. He didn't want me doing that, he said. He was fine. I was the one who was worried. His behavior was consistent with research on male partners' responses to their female partners' cancer.[69]

His caretaking reinforced some things I already knew about him, but in a way that made me feel like I was really seeing him for the first time. He cooked meals, came to any appointments I wanted him to attend, comforted me, laughed with me, went for drives with me, reminded me to have fun, fed me, loved me. I remember being extremely touched when he proudly told people that, even though I didn't feel well, I was walking every day. At the end of my treatment, we took off on a two-week road trip, which we dubbed the recovery road trip. He reminded me frequently during the trip that it wasn't the recoverED road trip, but the recoverY road trip, so I should go easy on myself. In a word, he was kind. I always knew this about him, but I realized during this time that he wanted nothing back. He just wanted me. No conditions, no expectations, and no keeping track of what he gave to me. I appreciate him and our relationship differently than I did before cancer. Everything was fine before cancer, so I'd happily go back to that time and never get cancer. But I can't. So I'll take the enhanced appreciation I have for my husband.

My appreciation for my husband doesn't mean that everything has been easy. We've had conversations we never dreamed we'd be having so early in life. I found myself asking him unimaginable things. I begged him to not put me in a box if I died, no matter how much it cost to deal with my body some other way. I asked him not to forget me. I made him promise to say my name. I was sometimes angry that he could not fully understand what I was experiencing. Who could, if they hadn't been through it? As with many women who undergo treatment for breast cancer, I have experienced changes in how I view my body and my sexual functioning. These changes have affected our relationship, although we've worked to maintain intimacy in the face of some really difficult moments.

I asked him to help me think through this part of the book by telling me how he thought cancer changed our relationship. He didn't have a lot to say about how our relationship changed during or after cancer, but what he did say made sense to me. The first thing was that we never really talked about cancer before, but now it's a part of our life every day. It's everywhere—we see it in movies, read it in books, hear about our friends getting it. And then there are all of the follow up appointments that continue even a decade after my initial treatment, so it's really never far from our minds. The second thing he commented on was sex. He said he's more cautious with me now than he was before. I understand that because I'm more cautious too. Chemo stopped my period and it never came back. Chemo and radiation affected and continue to affect my body, my body function, and my self-perception. In turn, they affect my relationship with my husband.

Couples find it difficult to discuss sexual changes. This is true in couples affected by both early stage and metastatic breast cancer. Sexual changes can be associated with depression, but talking in a mutually supportive, problem-solving way about sexual problems can help alleviate depressive symptoms.[70] Generally speaking, conversations about emotions as well as information-exchange are correlated with lower depressive symptoms for women with breast cancer, perhaps because both help the us make sense of our cancer.[71] The fact that talking about sexual problems is correlated with less depression doesn't make it easy. But it's worth trying.

Studies specifically about male partners of women with breast cancer are rare. One such study found that male partners are aware of their shifting roles in families, running the gamut from health management to family functioning.[72] In fact, the men in this study wanted to be involved in appointments, info-gathering, and decision making around their wives' cancer, while also trying to keep family life as normal as possible at home.

Cancer affects our family and family relationships beyond our spouses. There is not as much research on family relationships and cancer as there is on couples. One study found that family members of younger women with breast cancer take on new roles, including being present physically and emotionally, navigating the tension between needing help but not really wanting it, and serving as a buffer between the woman with breast cancer and her community.[73] In this same study, women both received support from and provided support to their families. One finding of family roles really hit home with me because my mother played such an important role in supporting me throughout my breast cancer experience: "Mothers of women with breast cancer played a pivotal role as support person that was both different and as important as spousal support;" whereas partners played the role of "protector," mothers wanted to "take away" their daughters' hurt.[74]

Women with advanced disease face some different family challenges than women with early-stage disease because the treatments and prognosis are often more extreme. The coping strategies of those of us with advanced disease and our caregivers are related to the mental quality of life for both. In one study that included a variety of caregivers (i.e., husbands, sisters, adult children, other family or friends), the communication-related coping strategies of providing emotional support, humor, and positive framing helped with quality of life. Non-communication coping strategies of religion and self-distraction also helped with quality of life. Venting, however, may negatively impact communication and stress, because it is doesn't promote interaction between family members. The kinds of coping strategies that both women and caregivers use correlate with the woman's level of symptoms and her quality of life.[75]

What I've come to realize is that my family relationships didn't really change much. Most continued to be what they already were—loving, close, detached, distant. I have a very close relationship with most of my immediate family (mother, father, brother, sister-in-law, niece), and a good relationship with most of my extended family (cousins, aunt, uncle, nieces, nephews, and others). I am not as close to my in-laws. I continued to experience that detachment during and since my cancer treatment, although some people occasionally checked in with my husband about how I was doing. My family relationships continued in ways I would have predicted.

My immediate family stepped toward me when I was sick, affirming our connections and offering support in myriad ways. They let me know they cared by calling me, and by sending candy from my hometown candy shop, cookies, a huge tin of crackers, cards, prayer shawls, prayers, gift cards, bubble bath. So many little things that told me they were thinking of me. These little things meant the world to me because they arrived at times when I felt alone, in the middle of waiting for the next chemotherapy treatment or slogging through the weeks of radiation.

They also did some big things. My brother Jeff talked to me a lot. I know he hated hearing me so sick, and he absolutely hates anything medical, but he listened to me through it all. He also never missed an opportunity to tell me that he loves me. My parents not only listened to me, but they also came to visit me, spending three weeks hanging out and helping around the house. My father told me he wished he could take the cancer instead of me, adopting the role of wanting to make the hurt go away. He also arrived for their visit with a shaved head in solidarity of my baldness. My mom hugged me and told me how good I looked. They were a great distraction in the middle of my chemotherapy treatment.

Friendships

Researchers recognize the importance of relational side effects across family and familial relationships. Many of my friendships also changed during and after my cancer diagnosis. My idea of what it means to be a friend also changed and that shift catalyzed many of the other changes. I became clear about the ways I was a friend to people and the ways others were friends to me. In a nutshell, I came to see that I was a go-to person for many people prior to cancer. I helped them with relational issues, work issues, and self issues. I liked the helper role and people came to expect me to perform it.

During cancer treatment, I simply could not be the helper friend that I once was. I was emotionally and physically exhausted. Most of my friends saw this long before I did and stepped toward me to help. They brought meals, sent cards, hung out with me, sent me my favorite kind of flannel pajamas, made me laugh, held me close. Some of the people who did these things were not even people I knew were my friends. They became my friends during the lowest part of my life. I was incredibly humbled and grateful for the people who supported me—and sometimes carried me—through the toughest moments of my life.

There were some friends and acquaintances who expected too

much from me, who didn't see the boundaries I had put in place, even after I had tried to make them clear. These friends called me with serious problems, asking me to help them solve them, without first assessing whether I was in a place to do so. (I liked it when people talked to me about their lives; I just couldn't always provide the depth of support they needed from me.) I got to the point of needing to be very explicit about my limits. For these friends, I simply told them that I needed to focus on myself and could not give them what they had become accustomed to getting from me.

There were two other friend responses that made me rethink some friendships. One was that some friends simply didn't show up for me. People who I had always thought were part of my friend circle never called to see how I was, never acknowledged my cancer, never reached out. I understand that cancer is hard to talk about and that it's hard to know what to say to people who have cancer. My husband suggested that some people just didn't know what to do, and that didn't make them bad people. I absolutely agree. These friends are not bad people, but they are not the kind of people I want in my life. I want people who step toward each other in times of crisis, even if they don't know what to say or do. Because showing up matters. The other kind of friend response that made me rethink friendships was what I considered inappropriate responses. This was uncommon, especially because I really did appreciate it if people responded at all. But there were a couple of instances when people echoed the idea that "everything happens for a reason" that troubled me. These moments revealed differences in our worldviews that caused me to distance myself, at least temporarily, from these friends.

I also found some friends in unexpected places. I found other women with breast cancer, some who had been diagnosed years ago and some who had been diagnosed when I was. These women were irreverent, funny, fierce, supportive, kind, and informative. I have tried to pay forward their surprising support of me by being there for other women with breast cancer. I found my breast cancer tribe with these women. These women got me in a way that most people couldn't.

I had always thought of friendship as reciprocal, and I have strived to give as good as I've received in my friendships. That some of my friendships were nonreciprocal was a surprise to me. I've also always thought of friendships as being based on core commonalities. That some of my friendships were not grounded in compatible worldviews surprised me. My father always told me that I'd be lucky if I could count my true friends on one hand. I still think I have more than five true friends, but I have definitely pruned my friendship network, and I don't easily add people to it. I am acutely aware that I only have so much energy and so much time in this world; I'm going to be judicious about where I spend both.

Summary

It takes an enormous amount of energy to deal with breast cancer. I didn't have the relational information presented in this chapter before or during my own treatment. I think it may well have overwhelmed me. I offer it to you as another resource in case you come up against relational challenges you need to address. In retrospect, I realize I didn't so much manage my relationships along the way as I trusted my gut and prioritized myself. My strongest, healthiest relationships were waiting for me when I emerged from treatment. Trust yourself.

Couple Communication Strategies

I offer communication strategies here with the explicit reminder that, although based in research on women with breast cancer and in my own experiences, these are things that may not work for you. You know your relationships best. Do what works for you.

Try to take a team approach by using "we" and "us" language instead of "you" and "I."
How you talk about yourselves in relation to your cancer can influence how you feel about yourselves as a couple.

Practice active listening skills.
By this, I mean try to see the conversation from your partner's perspective and check that you've understood where s/he is coming from before responding. This can be particularly important when talking about the more difficult conversational topics that a breast cancer diagnosis may bring—health care directives, end of life plans, sexual changes.

Encourage each other to talk to other people for support.
Your breast cancer is not a taboo subject.

Consider taking advantage of couples' interventions offered by your health center.
Whether it's counseling, support groups, or workshops, interventions can create moments to talk about difficult topics, improve coping and adjustment, and decrease distress.[76]

Try to talk openly about the tough topics (e.g., death, end of life plans, sex).
Bear in mind that time, place, and your partner's emotional state can influence how productive the conversations will be.

From my husband: Recognize that people express their fear and sorrow differently, both verbally and nonverbally.
This is consistent with some research that shows that women tend to talk more and to a broader range of people about their cancer than do their male partners, who talk mostly to their wives.[77]

Family Communication Strategies

I offer communication strategies here with the explicit reminder that, although based in research on women with breast cancer and in my own experiences, these are things that may not work for you. You know your relationships best. Do what works for you.

Consider having a family meeting.
Use this meeting to talk about your breast cancer so that family members can express their concerns and fears and perhaps take responsibility for part of your experience. This can reduce family stress because everyone has an opportunity to express themselves and to take an active role in your care.[78] It's also a great way to communicate your needs and share how your family can support you.

Include your adolescent and adult children in conversations about your cancer diagnosis, care, and prognosis.
Doing so can help everyone avoid unnecessary stress caused by information deficits. There isn't enough research on younger children for me to give you good guidance on including them in these conversations. My best advice is what I wrote in chapter 4: When you talk to children, give them information that is age appropriate and addresses how your cancer will affect them.

Extended Family and Friend Communication Strategies

I offer communication strategies here with the explicit reminder that, although based in research on women with breast cancer and in my own experiences, these are things that may not work for you. You know your relationships best. Do what works for you.

Understand that cancer may terrify family and friends.
Their responses may come from a place of fear.

Remember that it is not possible to get everything you need from one person.
Reach out to different people based on their skill sets.

Find your breast cancer tribe.
I found mine through a friend who connected me to the group of women I wrote about in this chapter. Your tribe may be quite similar to mine or starkly different from mine. The important thing is to find people who understand what you're experiencing.

Recognize that friendships sometimes have lifespans.
It's okay to let some friendships go. I find that I no longer bear the responsibility of calling people, making plans, and essentially nurturing my connections with as many people as I once did. The outcome for me has been a deepening of my core friendships and an enjoyment of my casual friendships without any of the stress I once experienced from trying to manage a larger network.

Decide how and with whom you want to spend your time and energy.
Ration your energy by being clear with family and friends if they are expecting too much from you, and by asking for help from people who make it easy.

Notes

Notes

Chapter 7:
When Everyone Else Thinks It's Over

Doctors and researchers recognize that people often feel adrift at the end of their initial treatment for cancer. By "initial treatment," I mean the intensive, first round of treatment for breast cancer, regardless of the stage of disease or the type of treatment. Endocrine therapy, treatment of recurrences, etc. are post-initial treatment. During my treatment, I felt like I had spent a long time in a small boat on a choppy lake, tethered to a secure dock. What I really wanted was to get to the other side of the lake. Once the tether was cut (i.e., initial treatment ended), I was still in the choppy water, but I was not tethered to anything anymore. No one was making sure I was okay, that I actually made it to the opposite shore. What I thought would be a moment of elation after treatment was actually a moment of intense anxiety for me. In this chapter, I discuss my experience post-treatment, comment on the words "survivor" and "survivorship," review some of the research on post-treatment communication challenges, and offer some communication strategies for dealing with life beyond initial breast cancer treatment.

Treatment Is Over—Shouldn't I Be Happy Now?

Treatment for breast cancer does not generally make a woman feel better, unlike treatment for many other illnesses, because we don't usually feel sick when we are diagnosed with breast cancer. I felt great when I was diagnosed, just having returned from a month-long vacation during which I helped host a celebration of my parents' 50 years of marriage. Life was good. However, after my lumpectomy and sentinel node biopsy, six rounds of chemotherapy, a dilation and curettage to rule out endometrial cancer, and 35 days of radiation, I was tired, bloated, weak, and burned. I lost my fingernails, had neuropathy, my eyes and nose watered unpredictably, and my brain felt foggy. And when my hair finally started to grow back, I had peach fuzz all over my face and neck. So, when people said things like, "But you're done now," or "It's all behind you," I wanted to scream. Or cry. I carried "it" with me everywhere. And it was heavy.

I think people were relieved that I was done with treatment. The thought that I might die terrified the people who love me, so it's not terribly surprising that the most common comment I heard was: "At least that's behind you now" or "It's all over" or "Time to get on with your life." Seriously? I certainly wasn't trying to milk the whole cancer experience, but did these people not understand that one of my chemotherapies was derived from mustard gas? I felt like crap physically and I felt completely depleted emotionally. But I was alive. Yes, I was thankful for that, but I also was angry and sad and depressed that I felt so miserable physically.

The day after my last radiation treatment, I sent the following email to my raggedy love army:

> *Good morning, my wonderful raggedy love army!*
>
> *This is my first official morning of life after cancer treatment. I dropped my car off at a body shop for some needed work, walked the mile or so home, stopped at Starbucks on the way, and am going to the University of Washington for a meeting in a little bit. How normal is all of that? I love it!*
>
> *If it's all the same to you, I'm not going to disband you. Although I'm hopeful that I won't have any more medical updates, I hear that the transition to a new normal can be, well, a transition. And I've come to rely on you a bit :) Thank you always.*
>
> *Love,*
> *Lisa*

Initially, I was elated. I was done. I had endured months of treatment, and I was ready to get back to my life. If I could have known then what I know now, I would have said, "Not so fast sister. You still have a lot to do." My cancer experience wasn't over; it just changed. Communication is an important part of this change, because "although life appears to return to normal on the surface, barriers to communication may diminish QOL [Quality of Life] for survivors by impeding the resolution of current or future problems."[79]

As I wrote in chapter 6, my cancer recovery started with a road trip. We had originally intended to go sit on a beach for a couple of weeks, but realized after a discussion with my oncologist, that I wasn't going to be able to be in the sun much after radiation. So we opted to jump into my convertible Miata and head to the national parks in southern Utah, making stops along the way to visit friends in Idaho, Utah, and Oregon. When we got to our first stop, we realized that the only planning we had done was where to stay. Neither of us knew anything about any of the parks. We hadn't done any research online; we hadn't purchased any guidebooks. Luckily, our national park going friends had come through with an itinerary for us, and we trusted them as we made our way from park to park.

I was surprised by my exhaustion, by my lack of stamina, by how easily my skin burned in the sun even with the sunblock I so religiously applied. Our trip was wonderful—the beauty, the relaxation, the togetherness—and it was also my first inkling that cancer wasn't quite done with me yet. It hadn't come back (in the sense of a recurrence), but the cancer experience was going to linger a lot longer than I had anticipated.

When we returned from our trip, I fully expected to be fully recovered. I remembered tentatively asking my radiation oncologist if she would mind extending my leave from work beyond the last day of my treatment, as I wanted to take some time to recover. She responded that she usually recommends that people take at least three additional weeks to recover. I assumed this meant that I would BE recovered three weeks after my last treatment. It took almost 2 years for me to feel mostly like myself again. Not quite my pre-cancer self, but close enough, and closer than I had dared hope a year before.

But I'm getting ahead of myself in my story. After our road trip, I went back to work until the end of the term, took the summer off (as I almost always did), and then returned to full time work the following fall. Just before spring term ended, my husband left for his yearly spring/summer fieldwork in the Bering Sea. My cancer diagnosis and initial treatment had conveniently fallen between his 2014 and 2015 trips. During the month or so he was gone, I usually did a bunch of house projects, reconnected with girlfriends, watched my favorite TV shows, and visited with my family in Massachusetts. The time alone was good for me. However, the 2015 trip was different.

After the elation of finishing treatment and the excitement of our road trip, I found myself in despair. Late one night, while sitting in bed with tears rolling down my face, I posted a plea for help to the women who had supported me through an online Facebook group. Once again, these women, most of whom I had never met, buoyed me. I wasn't alone. What I was feeling was normal. They recommended a book, *Dancing in Limbo*, pretty much the perfect response anyone could give to me.[80] They also had communication advice for me: I needed to educate the people around me that cancer doesn't end when initial treatment ends. So, I wrote the following email to my raggedy love army, who I needed just as much in that moment as I had ever needed them:

> *Hello my lovely raggedy love army,*
>
> *It's June, a year since my suspicious mammogram, a year since I visited my family in MA and then returned to Seattle to learn that I had cancer.*
>
> *Those are great words, aren't they: "I HAD cancer." Past tense.*
>
> *I am feeling healthy and I am slowly building my stamina. I've also learned that finishing treatment doesn't mean finishing the process of dealing with cancer. I've had a hard time adjusting back to regular life because very little seems regular... at the same time that*

everything looks just as I left it last July. Some people have encouraged me to let my community know that I still need them. So, here I am, letting you know that I still need you.

I realized that, during treatment, I put my head down and did what needed to be done. And now I'm processing it, probably long after most of you have processed that your wife/ daughter/sister/friend/ colleague/cousin/aunt/ relative had cancer. It's a bit of a gut punch to realize that I had cancer and that I still have to work through those three words: "I had cancer."

Thanks for hanging in with me while I find my new normal.

Love,
Lisa

I read the book *Dancing in Limbo.*[81] I explained how I was feeling to people. My mother, who seems to always get me, asked to read the book. She read it and then she took over some of the explaining for me. When people would say that "it is all behind you now," she would interject that it wasn't and she'd explain why. My love for her grew exponentially when she did that for me. I was tired and I was tired of explaining. She carried that load for me whenever she could and she supported me in carrying it when she couldn't.

My friends and doctors told me to expect it to take as long as my treatment lasted to feel good again once it was over. By my calculations, that meant that I should start feeling good again somewhere around January 2016. And I did. I was co-leading a study abroad program in Rome from January to March 2016, and that is where and when I started to feel like myself. I walked everywhere. I was astonished at my energy. My hair was starting to grow beyond the curly crew cut it had been for months. I was gaining physical ground daily. And I still needed my raggedy love army, as I told them in this email on 2/16/2016:

> *Hello my raggedy love army,*
>
> *I have been thinking about all of you a lot lately. A year ago, I was just about to start 7 weeks of daily radiation treatments. I had made it through surgery and chemotherapy.*
>
> *And now? Now, I'm in Rome, co-directing a study abroad program with my colleague. Dan is here with me too! We have 22 students; we're living in Rome; we're traveling around Europe; and we're living life.*
>
> *During my treatment, my friend Jessica told me that I was going to be able to do all the things I would have missed once treatment was over. And I am. And I am so incredibly grateful.*
>
> *I realize only now how sick I was last year. When I started back to work in earnest in September, I hobbled through the days. I made it; I did my job. But I was discouraged that I would not feel like me again. The doctors told me that it would take as long to heal from treatment as the treatment itself took. The magic number? 9 months. Nine months after my treatment ended, I landed in Rome. And, miraculously, my energy returned. Dan and I have been walking Rome like crazy. I feel more and more like myself. I think*

I'm back. Changed but back.

Since my last note to you, I've lost 2 friends to cancer and another has been diagnosed with cancer. They serve as reminders to me to live this day, to be joyful, to be grateful, to be alive.

I keep saying that this will be my last update, but obviously, I'm just kidding. I carry you with me still. Thank you.

Love,
Lisa

I also realized during this time, though, that I had reorganized my life priorities. I was so excited to be in Rome again, as I had to back out of a study abroad trip there when I was first diagnosed. But my patience was different than it had been. I loved the students (still do!), but I realized that I didn't want to be a disciplinarian. That wasn't my job. I'm a teacher. I wondered how this might translate into my work life when I returned to Seattle.

In the meantime, I awaited word on a sabbatical application I had submitted to write this book. With my sabbatical approved, I gained the luxury of time to figure out who I wanted to be at the University of Washington for the remainder of my career there. I know that I would not have applied for a full year if I hadn't gotten sick. It just wasn't my style. I wouldn't have thought I deserved it, and I would have been concerned that I would only receive partial pay for the year. But my priorities shifted during my cancer experience, and I took the whole year.

Part of my sabbatical mission was to regain my physical strength. Getting my body back in shape has been a difficult process. During treatment, I didn't think about what the surgeries, chemotherapies, and radiation were doing to my body long term. I knew they were beating me up short term, but I assumed (incorrectly) that my body would bounce back once initial treatment ended. I was wrong. Again. Chemotherapy attacks fast growing cells, regardless of whether they are cancerous. Muscle mass decreases significantly. Steroids help lessen the chemotherapy side effects, but also lead to puffiness. And radiation essentially cooks tissue. Like a fried egg. So that's all nice. I was weak, with little muscle mass, lots of fat, and some seriously damaged tissue. I also had other side effects that I've mentioned in other chapters, but these were the ones that slowed my progress toward strength. I got frustrated with my fatigue. I was unhappy with the way I looked. My skin was crepey. I had more visible cellulite. I had a chubby belly. My hands looked old. These were all pretty new to me.

I continued to walk after being in Rome. I was so inspired by the idea of walking more and more that I sold my car a year after I finished treatment so that I would be more apt to walk where I needed to go. My hope was that this would also allow me to slow my life down in all ways. On August 1, 2016, I joined a group fitness gym. My very first class was a barre class. I remember sweating a ton, and realizing, in the middle of class, that I had tears streaming down my face. But I was there. I couldn't do everything that I once could. I needed to take frequent breaks. But I kept going back. Five months later, I felt strong as I celebrated my 50th birthday in Belize, only to feel frustrated once again when I needed help back on the boat after a snorkeling trip. I was too weak to get back on the boat by myself.

When I asked my naturopath why I had such a tough time on the snorkeling trip, she asked me how long it had been since my treatment ended. I told her almost 2 years. She acknowledged that 2 years probably felt like a long time to me, but that it wasn't a long time in recovery. She encouraged me to keep going. I have. I work out 4-5 times each week, hiking and taking a variety of group fitness classes. Some days are easier than others, but I keep going. I see a difference in how my body looks and functions. My husband told me early on that he was impressed at how I persevered, even though for months and months there wasn't any real change in my body. I have to believe that there were invisible changes happening at a cellular level that finally became visible. I still sometimes get more tired than I'd like and I'm still not as strong as I once was, but I see glimpses of progress and I try to make the best of it.

Survivor

I'm called a survivor. I am in the survivorship phase of breast cancer. And yet I'm not comfortable with these words. I survivED breast cancer and breast cancer treatment, but the word "survivor" connotes something else to me. It sets up a dichotomy between those of us who are still alive and those of us who died. Survivors vs. what? "Failures?" "Losers?" Whether someone lives or dies after a breast cancer diagnosis has to do with a multitude of factors (e.g., access to healthcare, health insurance, socio-economic class, stage of diagnosis, tumor biology, etc.), including luck.

I think of myself as one of the lucky ones. That term suits me better. I am lucky. I didn't do anything brave or courageous or superhuman. I just got lucky. I was lucky to have my aggressive tumor detected through a mammogram. I was lucky to have a huge network of colleagues and friends who connected me with breast cancer experts around the country. I was lucky to have access to—and insurance that covers—topnotch cancer care. I was lucky to have the support of my family and friends. And, when it comes to still being alive, I was so incredibly lucky that my tumor responded to treatment. Because, when it comes right down to it, that's what differentiates those who live and those who die—the treatments available and our tumors' responses to it.

I'm not alone in feeling uncomfortable with the survivor label. The term "survivor" was coined in 1985 by Dr. Fitzhugh Mullan to reframe the idea of people with cancer as "victims."[82] The definition of survivor is fuzzy, ranging from characterizing people as survivors from the moment of diagnosis, to people who are disease free for a number of years, to including family members as survivors.[83] Recently, researchers have been concerned with finding out how women themselves feel about the survivor label.[84] They've found that women generally have a complicated relationship with the survivor label. Some embrace it; some reject it; others replace it with terms like "thriver" or "warrior;" while still others adopt it in ways that help them make sense of their experience. I fall into the rejection camp, after having tried unsuccessfully to adopt the term "thriver" as a replacement.

Our complex responses to the survivor label are rooted in our personal experiences with breast cancer and the cultural messages we get about what it means to be a survivor. Culturally, breast cancer survivors are portrayed as feminine, whole, and happy. Women whose personal experience of breast cancer aligns with this cultural model are likely more comfortable adopting the survivor label. However, for some, particularly those who fear recurrence, have a poor prognosis, or are physically disfigured, the term may be highly problematic.[85] A nuanced study of how women talk about the term survivor found that women might adopt or reject the term to varying degrees depending on how much they identify with other women with breast cancer, whether they feel they are cancer free, and how willing they are to adopt behavioral changes. In fact, we may change our feelings about the survivor label across contexts and time.[86]

Although it's a bit more cumbersome than the single word "survivor," I talk about myself as someone who had breast cancer. I'm choosing to use the past tense because I am NED (no evidence of disease). And honestly, it seems to make people feel more uncomfortable than I want to deal with when I say that I hope my breast cancer is gone. I still won't use the term survivor for myself. Language matters to me and this is my story. So, I had breast cancer.

Survivorship

Regardless of whether you embrace the survivor label, people will likely call you a survivor in medical contexts and you will likely be given some kind of survivorship care plan. Survivorship care plans provide women who have completed their initial breast cancer treatment with information about the treatment and its possible immediate and long-term health, social, and psychological impacts. The American Society of Clinical Oncology provides Survivorship Plan templates, which they update as new research about survivorship warrants. Here is a link to their most recent templates: https://www.asco.org/news-initiatives/current-initiatives/cancer-care-initiatives/prevention-survivorship/survivorship-compendium/care-planning.

The plan is also intended to be shared with our primary care physicians, as we transition from cancer care specialists back to regular health monitoring.[87] The label "survivorship" becomes problematic again at this point. Some women who complete their initial treatment for breast cancer live with stage 4 metastatic cancer as a chronic illness for the rest of their lives. Survivorship plans don't neatly fit their situation, and the label may discourage women from seeking the kind of information that both they and their primary care physicians need to monitor their health.

Given the problematic nature of the terms "survivor" and "survivorship," as well as the lack of consensus about what these terms mean in the research community, I define "survivor" as anyone who has finished their initial treatment for breast cancer, and "survivorship" as the phase that begins immediately following the initial treatment completion. Some researchers define the terms similarly, with "survivorship" as "the period following cessation of treatment"[88] and a survivor as "a person who has completed primary treatment for his/her cancer."[89]

Distinguishing between treatment and survivorship highlights the important, and often stressful, transition we make from initial treatment to the next phase of our experience. I use the terms "post-treatment" and "end of initial treatment" interchangeably, recognizing that many of us continue to be treated for breast cancer for the rest of our lives.

Survivorship and Communication

Just as communication plays a role in our relationship and personal well-being during initial treatment, it plays a role in our relationship and personal well-being during survivorship. Breast cancer survivors identify the development and maintenance of romantic relationships as a primary concern in survivorship.[90] Young breast cancer survivors, in particular, face challenges in establishing new relationships, relying on a pattern of relational development that includes disclosing their cancer and its physical manifestations to their potential partners early in their dating life.[91] For partnered women across age ranges, completing breast cancer treatment is yet another relationship turning point, where roles, responsibilities, and relational expectations need to be negotiated once again.[92]

Many survivors face changes in their sexuality and body image, both of which are tied not only to our sense of self, but also to our sense of relationships to others.[93] Young survivors experience significant body image disturbance, and related sexual and partner concerns.[94] As I mentioned in chapter 6, couples struggle in discussing sexual issues. With the end of treatment and the accompanying sense that life will go back to normal, sexual problems between couples can become exacerbated.

In addition to being a mechanism for addressing myriad relational changes, communication itself is associated with the physical and psychological well-being of breast cancer survivors. For instance, women who perceive that their family avoids communication about their cancer have worse mental health outcomes than women who perceive no family avoidance of talking about their cancer.[95] One study even found a connection between the quality of women's relationships and lower mortality or recurrence (although it's not really possible to determine whether the quality of the relationships actually affected the women's physical health or their good health affected the quality of their relationships).[96]

Breast cancer varies considerably from woman to woman. So too does our survivorship experience. With an increasing number of women living beyond an initial breast cancer experience, research on survivorship has increased, but not yet to the level of other aspects of breast cancer. As with much of the other research on breast cancer, most of the research participants in survivorship studies have been White, heterosexual, partnered, income-advantaged women. The existing research on women outside of this profile, then, warrants some attention here.

Culture, as I discussed in chapter 1, plays a role in how we think about and act in the world, including illness and the medical community. Women need more information about survivorship concerns (e.g., relationships, nutrition, emotions, sexuality) than we are generally given by healthcare providers, and minority women are sometimes given even less than other breast cancer patients.[97] In one study, African American breast cancer survivors identified post-treatment issues similar to the issues identified by women in the largely White population studies. Namely, they talked about (1) long-term physical side-effects of treatment, (2) the need for survivorship support, and (3) the centrality of emotional and psychological survivor concerns. These women also raised two unique issues: (1) the importance of their faith in their experience, and (2) a desire for support from an African American woman who had gone through breast cancer. Quality of life involves every aspect of our lives, but spirituality and religiosity are seldom studied in research on breast cancer survivors' quality of life. There were only 15 women in this study, so the generalizability of both similarities to and differences from other studies is not strong. These researchers call for more research on African American breast cancer survivors' quality of life that integrates physical, social, psychological, and spiritual well-being.[98]

Similarly, there are few studies on Asian American breast cancer survivors. One study found that Asian American survivors' quality of life was correlated with their own and their family members' general communication (i.e., not about cancer specifically) and their ability to reframe the cancer situation.[99] The women in this study, like the White women in many other studies, also experienced higher quality of life if they perceived their family communication as open. Interestingly, unlike findings about White women, Asian American survivors' quality of life was negatively impacted by their family members' solicitation of assistance from others, mostly likely due to cultural values of not imposing on others.

Another study echoed the cultural nuances of how we perceive support from others during our breast cancer experience. Chinese American women's acculturation (the degree to which a foreigner adapts to her host country) impacted their perceptions of the helpfulness of implicit, explicit, and tangible acts of support. Women who were less acculturated found implicit acts (e.g., companionship) and tangible acts (e.g., help with chores) more supportive; women who were more acculturated found explicit (e.g., emotional) acts more supportive. Cultural values influence the kinds of acts we find most supportive.[100]

Cultural influences also shape breast cancer survivors' experiences more generally. In one study, immigrant Latina breast cancer survivors identified cultural values that shaped their experience with breast cancer, including how they transitioned and then lived in the survivorship phase.[101] For example, as with African American women, the immigrant Latina women identified their faith in God as an important aspect of their ability to cope with cancer.

Even less is known about the breast cancer and survivor experiences of lesbian, bi-sexual, and transgender women. We need to learn more about the ways culture and our life histories shape our breast cancer experience from diagnosis to survivorship. While we wait for that research to occur, a larger study of low-income Latina, African American, and Asian American survivors reinforces the message with which I began this book: Communication is not going to cure our cancer, but it can empower us to maximize our interactions with our physicians, our families, and our communities.[102]

Summary

The end of the initial treatment for breast cancer looks different for everyone. For some, it really is the end of treatment. For most, there are lingering tests, scans, medications, and treatment side effects. For many, treatment continues for years. As with the other phases of your breast cancer experience, you get to define it and talk about it the way that works best for you. You may change your mind as you move further away from your diagnosis or transition to less medical surveillance and fewer medical interventions. The key is that it is your decision.

Communication Strategies

In the spirit of that empowerment, I offer here some strategies on how you might approach communication after your initial treatment ends.

Think about whether and how you want to be labeled, and how the label fits into your story.
Let other people know your choice and hold them to honoring it by repeating it as necessary.

Reach out to other people who have completed treatment.
It can be especially helpful to find someone who is like you in some ways, whether that be age, ethnicity, cancer profile, worldview, or something else that is meaningful to you. There are enough breast cancer survivors in the world that you are bound to find someone like you.

Educate yourself about what it means to be done with initial treatment, physically, mentally, relationally, and spiritually.

Educate your people about what it means to be done with initial treatment.
Tell your people about your post-treatment experience. Recommend the book, *Dancing in Limbo*.[103]

Talk to your partner about changes in your sexuality and body image.
Take advantage of resources and assistance from your healthcare center to support you as a couple during this time.[104]

Notes

Notes

Epilogue

I started this book project with the idea that I had something unique to offer other women experiencing breast cancer, because of my own experience and my expertise in communication. I hope that's true. But writing this book also had some unintended consequences. My psychiatrist suggested I write during my treatment, but I really didn't want to. Honestly, I didn't want to remember everything I was experiencing. She smiled a bit knowingly when I told her later that I was going to write a book. Writing about traumatic events like cancer can help people cope with these difficult life moments. Although after the fact, writing about my own cancer experience within the framework of the familiar topic of communication, has helped me cope. It has also been sad to revisit my experience, even so long after completing my initial treatment.

I've begun to put my experience in its place in my life story. I know it's not over, but I'm ready to move on. And now I must go out on our boat with my husband. And go out to dinner. Because that's what I do to remind myself that I have some living to do. I need to go do what I would have missed.

Endnotes

1 Bartlett, R. (1961). Cancer of the breast: Personal experience with 185 patients. *Annals of Surgery*, 154, 306-314.

2 O'Hair, H.D., Kreps, G.L., & Sparks, L.D. (2007). Conceptualizing cancer care and communication. In O'Hair, D., Kreps, G.L., & Sparks, L.D. (Eds.), *Handbook of communication and cancer care* (pp. 1-10), Hampton Press.

3 O'Hair, H.D., Kreps, G.L., & Sparks, L.D. (2007). Conceptualizing cancer care and communication. In O'Hair, D., Kreps, G.L., & Sparks, L.D. (Eds.), *Handbook of communication and cancer care* (pp. 1-10), Hampton Press.

4 Jatoi, I., Sung, H., & Jemal, A. (2022). The emergence of the racial disparity in U.S. breast-cancer mortality. *The New England Journal of Medicine*, 385(25), 2349-2352. https://doi.org/10.1056/NEJMp2200244

5 Gerend, M.A., & Pai, M. (2008). Social determinants of Black-White disparities in breast cancer mortality: A review. Cancer epidemiology, biomarkers & prevention, 17(11), 2913-2329. https://doi.org/10.1158/1055-9965.EPI-07-0633

Woods, L.M., Rachet, B., & Coleman, M. P. (2006). Origins of socio-economic inequalities in cancer survival: A review. *Annals of Oncology*, 17(1), 5–19. https://doi.org/10.1093/annonc/mdj007

6 Liu, Y., Malin, J.L., Diamant, A.L., Thind, A., & Maly, R.C. (2013). Adherence to adjuvant hormone therapy in low-income women with breast cancer: The role of provider-patient communication, *Breast Cancer Research and Treatment*, 137(3), 829-836.

7 Polacek, G.N.L.J., Ramos, M.C., & Ferrer, R.L. (2007). Breast cancer disparities and decision-making among U.S. women. *Patient Education and Counseling*, 65(2), 158–165. https://doi.org/10.1016/j.pec.2006.06.003

8 Thorne, S.E., Hislop, T.G., Armstrong, E., & Oglov, V. (2008). Cancer care communication: The power to harm and the power to heal? *Patient Education and Counseling*, 71(1), 35. https://doi.org/10.1016/j.pec.2007.11.010

9 Thorne, S.E., Hislop, T.G., Armstrong, E., & Oglov, V. (2008). Cancer care communication: The power to harm and the power to heal? *Patient Education and Counseling*, 71(1), 34-40. https://doi.org/10.1016/j.pec.2007.11.010

10 Robbins, M.L., López, A.M., Weihs, K.L., & Mehl, M.R. (2014). Cancer conversations in context: Naturalistic observation of couples coping with breast cancer. *Journal of Family Psychology*, 28(3), 380–390. https://doi.org/10.1037/a0036458

11 Lim, J. (2014). Communication, coping, and quality of life of breast cancer survivors and family/friend dyads: A pilot study of Chinese-Americans and Korean-Americans, *Psycho-oncology*, 23(11), 1243-1251. https://onlinelibrary.wiley.com/doi/10.1002/pon.3532

12 Lim, J. (2014). Communication, coping, and quality of life of breast cancer survivors and family/friend dyads: A pilot study of Chinese-Americans and Korean-Americans, *Psycho-oncology*, 23(11), 1243-1251. https://onlinelibrary.wiley.com/doi/10.1002/pon.3532

13 For an example of the interplay between individual and cultural narratives, see: Katriel, T., & Philipsen, G. (1981). "What we need is communication": "Communication" as a cultural category in some American speech. *Communication Monographs*, 48(4), 301–317. https://doi.org/10.1080/03637758109376064

14 altalang.com/beyond-words/fighting-an-illness-losing-a-battle/

15 bidenwhitehouse.archives.gov/cancermoonshot/

16 www.congress.gov/92/statute/STATUTE-85/STATUTE-85-Pg778-3.pdf

17 For more information about pinkwashing, take a look at breastcancer.org's article, breastcancer.org/about-breast-cancer/breast-cancer-awareness-month/pinkwashing

18 Ehrenreich, B. (2001, November). Welcome to Cancerland: A mammogram leads to a cult of pink kitsch, *Harper's Magazine*, 43-53.

19 DeShazer, M.K. (2013). *Mammographies: The cultural discourses of breast cancer narratives.* University of Michigan Press, 2. https://doi.org/10.3998/mpub.5571825

20 yaleglobal.yale.edu/content/treating-isis-cancer

21 medium.com/@joe_brewer/capitalism-has-a-metaphor-its-a-cancer-768baf05c942

22 humanvaluesinstitute.org/2433/message-16/

23 Frank, A.W. (2013). *The wounded storyteller: Body, illness, and metaphor* (2nd ed.). The University of Chicago Press.

24 Orgad, S. (2005). *Storytelling online: Talking breast cancer on the internet.* Peter Lang Publishing, Inc.

25 Mozen, P. (Director). (2018). *Life interrupted: Telling breast cancer stories* [Independent Film]. No Excuses Productions. https://www.lifeinterruptedfilm.com/

26 www.oed.com/dictionary/turning-point_n?tab=meaning_and_use#17188771

27 Mabaquiao, N. (2018). Speech act theory: From Austin to Searle. *Augustinian: A Journal for Humanities, Social Sciences, Business, and Education*, 19(1), 35-45.

28 Goffman, E. (1959). *The presentation of self in everyday life.* Doubleday & Company.

29 Matthews, A., Derlega, B., & Green, K. (2006). Self-disclosure in personal relationships. In *Cambridge Handbook of Personal Relationships*, 411.

30 Silk, S., & B. Goldman, B. (2013, April 7). How not to say the wrong thing. *LA Times* Op-Ed.

31 Hilton, B.A., Crawford, J.A., & Tarko, M.A. (2000). Men's perspectives on individual and family coping with their wives' breast cancer and chemotherapy. *Western Journal of Nursing Research*, 22(4), 438–459. https://doi.org/10.1177/019394590002200405

32 See, for example, the following two books:
Braddock, S.W., Kercher, J.M., Edney, J.J., Margaret, M., & Clark, M.M. (2015). *Straight talk about breast cancer: From diagnosis to recovery* (5th ed.). Addicus Books.

Port, E. (2015). *The new generation breast cancer book: How to navigate your diagnosis and treatment–and remain optimistic–in an age of information overload.* Ballantine Books.

33 Parker, P.A., Aaron, J., & Baile, W.F. (2008). Breast cancer: Unique communication challenges and strategies to address them. *The Breast Journal*, 15(1), 69. https://doi.org/10.1111/j.1524-4741.2008.00673.x

34 Street, R.L., Makoul, G., Arora, N.K., & Epstein, R.M. (2009). How does communication heal? Pathways linking clinician-patient communication to health outcomes. *Patient Education and Counseling*, 74(3), 295-301. https://doi.org/10.1016/j.pec.2008.11.015

35 Ha, J.F., & Longnecker, N. (2010). Doctor-patient communication: A review. *The Ochsner Journal*, 10(1), 38-43.

36 Ha, J.F., & Longnecker, N. (2010). Doctor-patient communication: A review. *The Ochsner Journal*, 10(1), 38.

37 Canzona, M.R., Garcia, D., Fisher, C.L., Raleigh, M., Kalish, V. & Ledford, C.J.W. (2016). Communication about sexual health with breast cancer survivors: Variation among patient and provider perspectives. *Patient Education and Counseling*, 99(11), 1814-1820. https://doi.org/10.1016/j.pec.2016.06.019

38 Martinez, K.A., Resnicow, K., Williams, G.C., Silva, M., Abrahamse, P., Shumway, D.A., Wallner, L.P., Katz, S.J., & Hawley, S.T. (2016). Does physician communication style impact patient report of decision quality for breast cancer treatment? *Patient Education and Counseling*, 99(12), 1947–1954. https://doi.org/10.1016/j.pec.2016.06.025

39 Vogel, B.A., Leonhart, R., & Helmes, A.W. (2009). Communication matters: The impact of communication and participation in decision making on breast cancer patients' depression and quality of life. *Patient Education and Counseling*, 77(3), 391–397. https://doi.org/10.1016/j.pec.2009.09.005

40 Shields, C.G., Ziner, K.W., Bourff, S.A., Schilling, K., Zhao, Q., Monahan, P., Sledge, G., & Champion, V. (2010). An intervention to improve communication between breast cancer survivors and their physicians. *Journal of Psychosocial Oncology*, 28(6), 610–629. https://doi.org/10.1080/07347332.2010.516811

41 Chen, J.Y., Tao, M.L., Tisnado, D., Malin, J., Ko, C., Timmer, M., Adams, J.L., & Ganz, P.A. (2008). Impact of physician-patient discussions on patient satisfaction. *Medical Care*, 46(11), 1157–1162. https://doi.org/10.1097/mlr.0b013e31817924bc

42 See, for example:
Volz, S., Moore, D.H., & Belkora, J.K. (2015). Do patients use decision and communication aids as prompted when meeting with breast cancer specialists? *Health Expectations: An International Journal of Public Participation in Health Care and Health Policy*, 18(3), 379–391. https://doi.org/10.1111/hex.12042

Brown, R.F., Bylund, C.L., Li, Y., Edgerson, S., & Butow, P. (2012). Testing the utility of a cancer clinical trial specific Question Prompt List (QPL-CT) during oncology consultations. *Patient Education and Counseling*, 88(2), 311–317. https://doi.org/10.1016/j.pec.2012.02.009

43 Venetis, M.K., Robinson, J.D., & Kearney, T. (2013). Consulting with a surgeon before breast cancer surgery: Patient question asking and satisfaction. *Journal of Health Communication*, 18(8), 943–959. https://doi.org/10.1080/10810730.2012.757391

44 Vogel, B.A., Leonhart, R., & Helmes, A.W. (2009). Communication matters: The impact of communication and participation in decision making on breast cancer patients' depression and quality of life. *Patient Education and Counseling*, 77(3), 391–397. https://doi.org/10.1016/j.pec.2009.09.005

45 Martinez, K.A., Resnicow, K., Williams, G.C., Silva, M., Abrahamse, P., Shumway, D.A., Wallner, L P., Katz, S J., & Hawley, S T. (2016). Does physician communication style impact patient report of decision quality for breast cancer treatment? *Patient Education and Counseling*, 99(12), 1947–1954. https://doi.org/10.1016/j.pec.2016.06.025

46 Hawkins, R P., Pingree, S., Shaw, B., Serlin, R.C., Swoboda, C., Han, J.Y., Carmack, C.L., & Salner, A. (2010). Mediating processes of two communication interventions for breast cancer patients. *Patient Education and Counseling*, 81(S1), S48–S53. https://doi.org/10.1016/j.pec.2010.10.021

47 Martinez, K.A., Resnicow, K., Williams, G.C., Silva, M., Abrahamse, P., Shumway, D.A., Wallner, L P., Katz, S J., & Hawley, S T. (2016). Does physician communication style impact patient report of decision quality for breast cancer treatment? *Patient Education and Counseling*, 99(12), 1947–1954. https://doi.org/10.1016/j.pec.2016.06.025

48 Siminoff, L.A., Graham, G.C., & Gordon, N.H. (2006). Cancer communication patterns and the influence of patient characteristics: Disparities in information-giving and affective behaviors. *Patient Education and Counseling*, 62(3), 355–360. https://doi.org/10.1016/j.pec.2006.06.011

49 Mott-Coles, S. (2014). Patients' cultural beliefs in patient-provider communication with African American women and Latinas diagnosed with breast cancer. *Clinical Journal of Oncology*, 18(4). 443-448. https://doi.org/10.1188/14.CJON.443-448

50 Kwan, M.L., Tam, E K., Ergas, I.J., Rehkopf, D H., Roh, J.M., Lee, M.M., Somkin, C. P., Stewart, A.L., & Kushi, L.H. (2013). Patient–physician interaction and quality of life in recently diagnosed breast cancer patients. *Breast Cancer Research and Treatment*, 139(2), 581–595. https://doi.org/10.1007/s10549-013-2569-z

51 Hull, S.J., Abril, E.P., Shah, D.V., Choi, M., Chih, M.-Y., Kim, S.C., Namkoong, K., McTavish, F., & Gustafson, D.H. (2016). Self-Determination Theory and computer-mediated support: Modeling effects on breast cancer patient's quality-of-life. *Health Communication*, 31(10), 1205–1214. https://doi.org/10.1080/10410236.2015.1048422

52 B Shields, C.G., Ziner, K.W., Bourff, S.A., Schilling, K., Zhao, Q., Monahan, P., Sledge, G., & Champion, V. (2010). An intervention to improve communication between breast cancer survivors and their physicians. *Journal of Psychosocial Oncology*, 28(6), 610–629. https://doi.org/10.1080/07347332.2010.516811

53 Parker, P.A., Aaron, J., & Baile, W.F. (2008). Breast cancer: Unique communication challenges and strategies to address them. *The Breast Journal*, 15(1), 69. https://doi.org/10.1111/j.1524-4741.2008.00673.x

54 Martinez, K.A., Resnicow, K., Williams, G.C., Silva, M., Abrahamse, P., Shumway, D.A., Wallner, L.P., Katz, S.J., & Hawley, S T. (2016). Does physician communication style impact patient report of decision quality for breast cancer treatment? *Patient Education and Counseling*, 99(12), 1947–1954. https://doi.org/10.1016/j.pec.2016.06.025

55 Baxter, L.A., & Bullis, C. (1986). Turning points in developing romantic relationships. *Human Communication Research*, 12(4), 469–493. https://doi.org/10.1111/j.1468-2958.1986.tb00088.x

56 Weber, K.M., & Solomon, D.H. (2008). Locating relationship and communication issues among stressors associated with breast cancer. *Health Communication*, 23(6), 548–559. https://doi.org/10.1080/10410230802465233

57 Rottmann, N., Hansen, D.G., Larsen, P.V., Nicolaisen, A., Flyger, H., Johansen, C., & Hagedoorn, M. (2015). Dyadic coping within couples dealing with breast cancer: A longitudinal, population-based study. *Health Psychology*, 34(5), 486–495. https://doi.org/10.1037/hea0000218

58 Manne, S.L., Siegel, S., Kashy, D., & Heckman, C.J. (2014). Cancer-specific relationship awareness, relationship communication, and intimacy among couples coping with early-stage breast cancer. *Journal of Social and Personal Relationships*, 31(3), 314–334. https://doi.org/10.1177/0265407513494950

59 Manne, S.L., Siegel, S., Kashy, D., & Heckman, C.J. (2014). Cancer-specific relationship awareness, relationship communication, and intimacy among couples coping with early-stage breast cancer. *Journal of Social and Personal Relationships*, 31(3), 316. https://doi.org/10.1177/0265407513494950

60 Yu, Y., & Sherman, K.A. (2015). Communication avoidance, coping and psychological distress of women with breast cancer. *Journal of Behavioral Medicine*, 38(3), 567. https://doi.org/10.1007/s10865-015-9636-3

61 See: Goldsmith, D.J., Miller, L.E., & Caughlin, J.P. (2007). Openness and avoidance in couples communicating about cancer. *Annals of the International Communication Association*, 31(1), 62–115.

62 Hague, K.E., Martinez, M.A., & Robbins, M.L. (2024). Qualitative analysis of naturalistically observed conversations among same- and different-gender couples coping with breast cancer. *Personal Relationships*, 31(3), 758–775. https://doi.org/10.1111/pere.12558

63 Hague, K.E., Martinez, M.A., & Robbins, M.L. (2024). Qualitative analysis of naturalistically observed conversations among same- and different-gender couples coping with breast cancer. *Personal Relationships*, 31(3), 758–775. https://doi.org/10.1111/pere.12558

64 See, for example:
Skerrett, K. (1998). Couple adjustment to the experience of breast cancer. *Families, Systems & Health*, 16(3), 281–298. https://doi.org/10.1037/h0089855

Li, Q., & Loke, A.Y. (2014). A literature review on the mutual impact of the spousal caregiver–cancer patients dyads: 'Communication,' 'reciprocal influence,' and 'caregiver–patient congruence.' *European Journal of Oncology Nursing: The Official Journal of European Oncology Nursing Society*, 18(1), 58–65. https://doi.org/10.1016/j.ejon.2013.09.003

65 Skerrett, K. (1998). Couple adjustment to the experience of breast cancer. *Families, Systems & Health*, 16(3), 281–298. https://doi.org/10.1037/h0089855

66 Yu, Y., & Sherman, K.A. (2015). Communication avoidance, coping and psychological distress of women with breast cancer. *Journal of Behavioral Medicine*, 38(3), 573. https://doi.org/10.1007/s10865-015-9636-3

67 Donovan-Kicken, E., & Caughlin, J.P. (2010). A multiple goals perspective on topic avoidance and relationship satisfaction in the context of breast cancer. *Communication Monographs*, 77(2), 231–256. https://doi.org/10.1080/03637751003758219

68 Pistrang, N., Barker, C., & Rutter, C. (1997). Social support as conversation: Analysing breast cancer patients' interactions with their partners. *Social Science & Medicine* (1982), 45(5), 773–782. https://doi.org/10.1016/S0277-9536(96)00413-3

69 Segrin, C., Badger, T., Sieger, A., Meek, P., & Lopez, A.M. (2006). Interpersonal well-being and mental health among male partners of women with breast cancer. *Issues in Mental Health Nursing*, 27(4), 371–389. https://doi.org/10.1080/01612840600569641

70 Milbury, K., & Badr, H. (2013). Sexual problems, communication patterns, and depressive symptoms in couples coping with metastatic breast cancer. *Psycho-Oncology* (Chichester, England), 22(4), 814–822. https://doi.org/10.1002/pon.3079

71 Robbins, M.L., López, A.M., Weihs, K.L., & Mehl, M.R. (2014). Cancer conversations in context: Naturalistic observation of couples coping with breast cancer. *Journal of Family Psychology*, 28(3), 380–390. https://doi.org/10.1037/a0036458

72 Hilton, B.A., Crawford, J.A., & Tarko, M.A. (2000). Men's perspectives on individual and family coping with their wives' breast cancer and chemotherapy. *Western Journal of Nursing Research*, 22(4), 438–459. https://doi.org/10.1177/019394590002200405

73 Coyne, E., Wollin, J., & Creedy, D.K. (2012). Exploration of the family's role and strengths after a young woman is diagnosed with breast cancer: Views of women and their families. *European Journal of Oncology Nursing: The Official Journal of European Oncology Nursing Society*, 16(2), 124–130. https://doi.org/10.1016/j.ejon.2011.04.013

74 Coyne, E., Wollin, J., & Creedy, D.K. (2012). Exploration of the family's role and strengths after a young woman is diagnosed with breast cancer: Views of women and their families. *European Journal of Oncology Nursing: The Official Journal of European Oncology Nursing Society*, 16(2), 128. https://doi.org/10.1016/j.ejon.2011.04.013

75 Kershaw, T., Northouse, L., Kritpracha, C., Schafenacker, A., & Mood, D. (2004). Coping strategies and quality of life in women with advanced breast cancer and their family caregivers. *Psychology & Health*, 19(2), 139–155. https://doi.org/10.1080/08870440310001652687

76 Regan, T.W., Lambert, S.D., Girgis, A., Kelly, B., Kayser, K., & Turner, J. (2012). Do couple-based interventions make a difference for couples affected by cancer?: A systematic review. *BMC Cancer*, 12(1), Article 279. https://doi.org/10.1186/1471-2407-12-279

77 Robbins, M.L., López, A.M., Weihs, K.L., & Mehl, M.R. (2014). Cancer conversations in context: Naturalistic observation of couples coping with breast cancer. *Journal of Family Psychology*, 28(3), 380–390. https://doi.org/10.1037/a0036458

78 Weber, K.M., & Solomon, D.H. (2008). Locating relationship and communication issues among stressors associated with breast cancer. *Health Communication*, 23(6), 548–559. https://doi.org/10.1080/10410230802465233

79 Bloom, J.R., Stewart, S.L., D'Onofrio, C.N., Luce, J., & Banks, P.J. (2008). Addressing the needs of young breast cancer survivors at the 5 year milestone: Can a short-term, low intensity intervention produce change? *Journal of Cancer Survivorship*, 2(3), 190–204. https://doi.org/10.1007/s11764-008-0058-x

80 Halvorson-Boyd, G., & Hunter, L. (1995). *Dancing in limbo: Making sense of life after cancer*. Jossey-Bass Publishers. https://www.loc.gov/catdir/toc/onix07/95009135.html

81 Halvorson-Boyd, G., & Hunter, L. (1995). *Dancing in limbo: Making sense of life after cancer*. Jossey-Bass Publishers. https://www.loc.gov/catdir/toc/onix07/95009135.html

82 Kaiser, K. (1982). The meaning of the survivor identity for women with breast cancer. *Social Science & Medicine*, 67(1), 79-87. https://doi.org/10.1016/j.socscimed.2008.03.036

83 Jagielski, C.H., Hawley, S.T., Corbin, K., Weiss, M.C., & Griggs, J.J. (2012). A phoenix rising: Who considers herself a "survivor" after a diagnosis of breast cancer? *Journal of Cancer Survivorship*, 6(4), 451–457. https://doi.org/10.1007/s11764-012-0240-z

84 See, for example:
Jagielski, C.H., Hawley, S.T., Corbin, K., Weiss, M.C., & Griggs, J.J. (2012). A phoenix rising: Who considers herself a "survivor" after a diagnosis of breast cancer? *Journal of Cancer Survivorship*, 6(4), 451–457. https://doi.org/10.1007/s11764-012-0240-z

Kaiser, K. (1982). The meaning of the survivor identity for women with breast cancer. *Social Science & Medicine*, 67(1), 79-87. https://doi.org/10.1016/j.socscimed.2008.03.036

Stephenson, W.H., Fletcher, P.C., & Schneider, M.A. (2013). Women with breast cancer: Embracing and distancing themselves from the term cancer survivor. *Clinical Nursing Studies*, 2(1). https://doi.org/10.5430/cns.v2n1p64

85 Kaiser, K. (1982). The meaning of the survivor identity for women with breast cancer. *Social Science & Medicine*, 67(1), 79-87. https://doi.org/10.1016/j.socscimed.2008.03.036

86 Stephenson, W.H., Fletcher, P.C., & Schneider, M.A. (2013). Women with breast cancer: Embracing and distancing themselves from the term cancer survivor. *Clinical Nursing Studies*, 2(1). https://doi.org/10.5430/cns.v2n1p64

87 Todd, B.L., Feuerstein, M., Gehrke, A., Hydeman, J., & Beaupin, L. (2015). Identifying the unmet needs of breast cancer patients post-primary treatment: The Cancer Survivor Profile (CSPro). *Journal of Cancer Survivorship*, 9(2), 137–160. https://doi.org/10.1007/s11764-015-0428-0

88 Keesing, S., Rosenwax, L., & McNamara, B. (2016). A dyadic approach to understanding the impact of breast cancer on relationships between partners during early survivorship. *BMC Women's Health*, 16(1), Article 57, 2. https://doi.org/10.1186/s12905-016-0337-z

89 Mollica, M., & Nemeth, L. (2015). Transition from patient to survivor in African American breast cancer survivors. *Cancer Nursing*, 38(1), 17. https://doi.org/10.1097/NCC.0000000000000120

90 Miller, L.E. (2015). Young breast cancer survivors' experiences of uncertainty. *Journal of Applied Communication Research*, 43(4), 429–449. https://doi.org/10.1080/00909882.2015.1083600

91 Kurowecki, D., & Fergus, K.D. (2014). Wearing my heart on my chest: Dating, new relationships, and the reconfiguration of self-esteem after breast cancer. *Psycho-Oncology* (Chichester, England), 23(1), 52–64. https://doi.org/10.1002/pon.3370

92 Miller, L.E. (2015). Young breast cancer survivors' experiences of uncertainty. *Journal of Applied Communication Research*, 43(4), 429–449. https://doi.org/10.1080/00909882.2015.1083600

Keesing, S., Rosenwax, L., & McNamara, B. (2016). A dyadic approach to understanding the impact of breast cancer on relationships between partners during early survivorship. *BMC Women's Health*, 16(1), Article 57. https://doi.org/10.1186/s12905-016-0337-z

93 Pelusi, J. (2006). Sexuality and body image: Research on breast cancer survivors documents altered body image and sexuality. *The American Journal of Nursing*, 106(3 Suppl), 32–38. https://doi.org/10.1097/00000446-200603003-00013

94 Paterson, C.L., Lengacher, C.A., Donovan, K.A., Kip, K.E., & Tofthagen, C.S. (2016). Body image in younger breast cancer survivors: A systematic review. *Cancer Nursing*, 39(1), E39–E58. https://doi.org/10.1097/NCC.0000000000000251

95 Mallinger, J.B., Griggs, J.J., & Shields, C.G. (2006). Family communication and mental health after breast cancer. *European Journal of Cancer Care*, 15(4), 355–361. https://doi.org/10.1111/j.1365-2354.2006.00666.x

96 Epplein, M., Zheng, Y., Zheng, W., Chen, Z., Gu, K., Penson, D., Lu, W., & Shu, X.-O. (2011). Quality of life after breast cancer diagnosis and survival. *Journal of Clinical Oncology*, 29(4), 406–412. https://doi.org/10.1200/JCO.2010.30.6951

[97] Mollica, M., & Nemeth, L. (2015). Transition from patient to survivor in African American breast cancer survivors. *Cancer Nursing*, 38(1), 16–22. https://doi.org/10.1097/NCC.0000000000000120

[98] Mollica, M., & Nemeth, L. (2015). Transition from patient to survivor in African American breast cancer survivors. Cancer Nursing, 38(1), 16–22. https://doi.org/10.1097/NCC.0000000000000120

[99] Lim, J. (2014). Communication, coping, and quality of life of breast cancer survivors and family/friend dyads: A pilot study of Chinese-Americans and Korean-Americans. *Psycho-Oncology* (Chichester, England), 23(11), 1243–1251. https://doi.org/10.1002/pon.3532

[100] Wong, C. C. Y., & Lu, Q. (2017). Match between culture and social support: Acculturation moderates the relationship between social support and well-being of Chinese American breast cancer survivors. *Quality of Life Research*, 26(1), 73–84. https://doi.org/10.1007/s11136-016-1362-y

[101] Lopez-Class, M., Perret-Gentil, M., Kreling, B., Caicedo, L., Mandelblatt, J., & Graves, K.D. (2011). Quality of life among immigrant Latina breast cancer survivors: Realities of culture and enhancing cancer care. *Journal of Cancer Education*, 26(4), 724–733. https://doi.org/10.1007/s13187-011-0249-4

[102] Maly, R.C., Liu, Y., Liang, L., & Ganz, P.A. (2015). Quality of life over 5 years after a breast cancer diagnosis among low-income women: Effects of race/ethnicity and patient-physician communication. *Cancer*, 121(6), 916–926. https://doi.org/10.1002/cncr.29150

[103] Halvorson-Boyd, G., & Hunter, L. (1995). *Dancing in limbo: Making sense of life after cancer*. Jossey-Bass Publishers. https://www.loc.gov/catdir/toc/onix07/95009135.html

[104] Keesing, S., Rosenwax, L., & McNamara, B. (2016). A dyadic approach to understanding the impact of breast cancer on relationships between partners during early survivorship. *BMC Women's Health*, 16(1), Article 57. https://doi.org/10.1186/s12905-016-0337-z

www.ingramcontent.com/pod-product-compliance
Lightning Source LLC
LaVergne TN
LVHW022225200926
848481LV00006B/2120